Primary Sources for the History of Pharmacy in the United States

A SELECTION OF PRIMARY SOURCES FOR THE HISTORY OF PHARMACY IN THE UNITED STATES

Books and Trade Catalogs From the Colonial Period to 1940

By Nydia M. King, Ph.D.
Professor of History of Pharmacy (Retired)
University of Puerto Rico

American Institute of the History of Pharmacy
located at the University of Wisconsin-Madison
Madison ◆ 1987

Publication No. 9
Gregory J. Higby and Elaine C. Stroud, General Editors

A Fischelis Publication
on Recent History and Trends of Pharmacy

second of a series aided by a fund established
in the American Institute of the History of Pharmacy

by

ROBERT P. FISCHELIS (1891–1981)

pharmacist · administrator · author · educator

SAMPLE ENTRY

C27[1]Y<small>OUNGKEN</small>, Heber W[ilkinson][2], 1885–1963

A textbook of pharmacognosy.[3] Philadelphia: P. Blakiston's Son & Co.[4], [c. 1921][5].1 l^6, v–x, 1 l^6, 3–538 p. 15×23[7] cm. (Evans 24014)[8] (DNLM)[9] **AIHP 85**[10]

1. Entry number.
2. Author names in some entries are in more complete form than on the titlepages of original sources.
3. Titles are shown in lower case except for the first word and proper nouns, regardless of the printed style on the original titlepages.
4. Names of publishers are given exactly as they appear on the titlepages.
5. When no date appears on the original titlepage, an approximate date is given in brackets, usually either the copyright date or the date on the preface.
6. The number of unnumbered leaves in the copy examined (in this example "1 l " = one leaf).
7. Dimensions of the cover on the copy examined.
8. Evans catalog number.
9. Library location (abbreviation) of cited work.
10. University Microfilms International catalog number.

Abbreviations List

AIHP	American Institute of the History of Pharmacy
PPAmP	American Philosophical Society Library, Philadelphia
ICRL	Center for Research Libraries, Chicago
OCLloyd	Lloyd Library, Cincinnati
MBCP	Massachusetts College of Pharmacy Library, Boston
DNLM	National Library of Medicine, Washington, D.C.
WU	University of Wisconsin Libraries, Madison

FACSIMILE EDITIONS AVAILABLE

This booklet is intended as a handy guide to representative works drawn from various categories of pharmaceutical literature in various periods of the history of the United States. It likewise serves as a key to, and an interpretation of, the facsimile editions that have been issued to make the works readily available once more. Of the eighty-nine out-of-print works cited in this booklet, eighty-five are available as facsimile editions; Wood and LaWall, *United States Dispensatory* (A6, WU), Peter Smith, *Indian Doctor's Dispensatory* (C28, OCLloyd), Torald Sollman, *A Manual of Pharmacology* (C34, WU), and John Day & Co., *Catalogue of Drugs* (D1, PPAmP) are the exceptions. To implement this two-phase project the American Institute of the History of Pharmacy invited Nydia M. King, retired professor at the University of Puerto Rico, to undertake the historical and bibliographical work and invited University Microfilms International to produce and distribute the facsimile editions.

Readers may purchase the complete text of eighty-five of the works discussed in this booklet (see paragraph above for the titles that are not included), either as a microfiche collection or as selected individual softbound volumes.

For additional information, inquire about "Primary Sources in the History of Pharmacy" at: Research Collections, University Microfilms International, 300 North Zeeb Road, Ann Arbor, MI 48106. For information by telephone, contact an Account Representative of UMI Research Collections toll-free at 800-423-6108. In Michigan, Alaska, and Hawaii, call collect, 313-761-4700. In Canada, call toll-free at 800-343-5299 or Telex (230) 23-5569. Canadians also may access information through "Envoy 100" and "OnTyme" services.—*The American Institute of the History of Pharmacy.*

CONTENTS

Foreword   ix

Introduction   xi

Acknowledgements   xv

**Part One: Categorical List of Selected Works
   with Descriptive Essays   1**
A. Dispensatories   1
B. Pharmacopoeias and Formularies   8
C. Textbooks and Reference Books   24
   Pharmacy
   Materia Medica, Pharmacognosy, Pharmacology and
      Therapeutics
   Pharmaceutical Chemistry
   Laws and Regulations
   Other Books: Proceedings, Surveys, Yearbooks, Studies
D. Trade Catalogs   83

Part Two: Chronological List of Works by Publication Dates   91

Part Three: Alphabetical List of Works by Authors   107

FOREWORD

One day early in 1983 a phone call from Rio Piedras came to me as the Director of the American Institute of the History of Pharmacy. It was Professor Nydia M. King of the University of Puerto Rico, who had just finished her term as the first woman President of the AIHP. Her restless energy always had been a hallmark, and now she was eager to do something more for the Institute—something historical, but not too large scale. After discussing several possibilities, Professor King decided to do what I had hoped all along she would do: undertake the booklet now before us.

The concept grew out of an ambition we harbored in the Institute: to characterize and reproduce in facsimile a core literature drawn from the American pharmaceutical past, works that had become hard to find. Even the pharmaceutical collections at many universities had been weakened historically through overzealous pruning of the holdings over the decades. This paucity of sources often handicaps serious teaching and research in pharmacy's history at colleges of pharmacy. A mandate that seemed tailor-made to help repair this gap in literature sources came in September that year when the AIHP Council established and funded an annual program "to upgrade historical resources at universities in the United States teaching the history of pharmacy."

With support thus assured, we set to work with renewed enthusiasm to formulate the project that here comes to fruition. The author worked in the collections at Madison and Bethesda for three summers, at her own expense it should be said (except for one transportation grant from the AIHP). A tentative draft of the booklist was out of the typewriter by the fall of 1983, when we had our first conference with representatives of University Microfilms International. Through their fine cooperation all but a few of the works discussed by Professor King will remain permanently available from UMI both as microfiche and as hard copy bound volumes. It merits recognition that Anita L. Werling and Sally Scarnecchia, two principals of the firm's Research Collections division, never lost their enthusiasm for the historical significance of the project even when its limited commercial appeal became obvious.

Still more it has been a pleasure to be associated with the author during the several stages of the project and to observe at first hand the time and talent Nydia King so generously invested. The selection process alone was forbidding: to sift fewer than a hundred representative works out of the many hundreds published during the evolution of American pharmacy, then to characterize each work

ix

and its author for the reader. Unlike similar projects in other fields, it has not been Professor King's aim to present the "great books" or "milestone" volumes of pharmacy. Rather she shows us how pharmacy has been and came to be by taking us back to the bedrock of primary sources that represent different categories of pharmaceutical literature and different stages of American pharmacy's history. In this way she has made a contribution that will endure in usefulness.

—Glenn Sonnedecker

Madison, Wisconsin

INTRODUCTION

The literature of pharmacy mirrors, however imperfectly, the state of the profession at a given time. The bedrock of this literature consists of the volumes that helped to guide pharmaceutical studies and activities in their time and that now serve as primary sources for the history of pharmacy. The booklet I have prepared characterizes the content and the authors of eighty-nine volumes selected as representative of various categories and periods of American pharmaceutical literature. These works either were written and published in the United States or were reprinted here from European works (sometimes modified to suit American conditions, sometimes not). They offer us a first-hand glimpse of the state of knowledge and practice in cross-sections of history, ranging from Colonial times to 1940. The 1940 terminus is not entirely arbitrary: It was a time of renewal in American pharmaceutical literature, turning on striking changes in the level of pharmaceutical science and increasing specialization of literature. Moreover, a majority of the works published since then are still in print or at least readily available in libraries.

In contrast, all of the works here discussed are out of print and hard to find. Therefore my purpose has been not only to provide a highly selective guide to representative sources but to define the scope of a project of facsimile editions—an objective set by the American Institute of the History of Pharmacy—which will make the content of these volumes widely available once more. The choice of titles was bound to be somewhat arbitrary. The main objective has been to represent or typify various types of pharmaceutical literature, whether imposing pharmacopoeias or modest trade catalogs. There was no over-riding concern to select always the "milestone" or "pioneering" works in the service of pharmacy. First editions have been cited except when a later edition was appropriate to help represent a later period, or was appropriate for another reason cited in the following essays.

The titles listed and discussed were selected from among about twice as many volumes that resulted from a preliminary screening of the literature (drawn not only from the literature of "regular" practice, but Thomsonian, homeopathic, and eclectic). Each volume was examined in terms of any of the following criteria: effective representation of the practice and development of the profession and science of American pharmacy; potential as a primary source for writing or teaching the history of specific or general pharmaceutical topics, or for representing particular classes of the pharmaceutical literature; the reputation of the authors; and the influence on other works.

This booklet is in three parts. In the *first part* the volumes are classified into four categories: A. Dispensatories, B. Pharmacopoeias and Formularies, C. Textbooks and Reference Books, and D. Trade Catalogs. Within each category (except Trade Catalogs) the reader finds for each book listed a verified bibliographic citation, a short essay defining the character and historical significance of the volume and offering a biographical vignette of the author and references to comparable works. The section on trade catalogs begins with a general introduction explaining the place of these publications in the pharmaceutical literature and their value as historical sources. The individual catalogs are then described briefly to indicate their scope and special features.

The *second part* of the booklet offers an overall view of the books from all categories within specified time-periods by listing them chronologically by date of publication. The *third part* presents the titles in alphabetic order by authors and serves as an index to the essays.

Overview of the Selected Sources

British dispensatories and pharmacopoeias influenced greatly the establishment of the literature of American pharmacy. From the seventeenth century, dispensatories commonly combined an English translation (from the Latin) of a pharmacopoeia with commentaries and other material, thus becoming more practical than the pharmacopoeia as such. These dispensatories were popular among both medical practitioners, and among independent preparers and dispensers of medicines. It is not surprising, then, that the first known medical book published in United States territory and the first book of importance in the rise of the American medico-pharmaceutical literature were both dispensatories. The present listing and the separate facsimile editions include these two books (A1 and A2) and four other representative works of this class.

American guidebooks for the preparation of medicines—pharmacopoeias and formularies—began appearing in the late eighteenth and early nineteenth centuries, with roots in their British counterparts. Sixteen books presented here are editions of the official compendia, of their precursors, and of authoritative or popular works supplementary to them.

Over half of the volumes here characterized are textbooks and reference works classified as (1) Pharmacy; (2) Materia Medica, Pharmacognosy, Pharmacology and Therapeutics; (3) Pharmaceutical Chemistry; (4) Laws and Regulations; and (5) Other Books, which include proceedings, surveys, yearbooks, and reports of studies.

Pharmacy textbooks published or authored in the United States did not appear until the middle of the nineteenth century, reflecting the fact that the British pharmaceutical literature began to flourish after the 1840s, and that American pharmacy generally mirrored the British model. The first textbook was prompted by the keenly felt need for an English-language textbook when a separate pharmacy course was established at the Philadelphia College of Pharmacy (1846). Also represented are the early elementary and practical textbooks, the encyclopedic and the scientific-informative reference works, the specialized volumes (published later), a pharmaceutical dictionary, and a tract on homeopathic pharmaceutics.

For many years the term "materia medica" embraced everything related to medicinal substances, but eventually the subject matter branched into separate disciplines, notably pharmacy, pharmacognosy, pharmacology and therapeutics. Books bearing the ancient collective title were still on the scene in the United States—concurrently with some dispensatories, pharmacopoeias, formularies, and trade catalogs—long before pharmacy books *per se* appeared. The twenty-three books depicted in this materia medica section are American works on simple and compound medicinals, indigenous medicinal plants, and homeopathic materia medica; works on the classification and action of drugs, and early pharmacognosy and pharmacology textbooks.

With a European tradition behind it, chemistry applied to pharmacy was one of two subjects in early American pharmaceutical education—the other being the combination of materia medica and pharmacy. British texts or their American editions were exclusively used as textbooks until at least the 1870s when the first such books written in the United States began to appear. Five landmark editions are presented here, including books on general pharmaceutical chemistry, the detection of drug adulteration, determination of identity and quality, pharmaceutical assaying (alkaloid standardization), and biostandardization of drugs.

Pharmacy-related regulations began to appear in the United States early in the nineteenth century. Local attempts at some kind of control of the practice of pharmacy were made in such cities as New Orleans (1804), New York (1832), and Louisville, Kentucky (1851); and state-wide attempts in four southern states provided for the licensing of pharmacists, but as part of the regulation of medicine. The custom of setting standards for pharmacy practice by means of separate state statutes was established later in the century. Most of the first state pharmacy laws—at least forty by the 1890s—followed a model law prepared in 1869 by a committee of the American Pharmaceutical Association. Later statutes often were based on an updated draft adopted by the Association in 1900. These two model drafts provided the pattern and main features of today's pharmacy laws.

State regulations pertaining to the sale of poisons and adulterated drugs also date back to the 1800s, either as clauses in the first state pharmacy laws or as separate statutes. By the end of the century the need for national (federal) control of the interstate drug supply was obvious. But it was not until the early twentieth century that sweeping federal drug laws were enacted—the Food and Drug Act of 1906 and the Food, Drug and Cosmetic Act of 1938. These laws, although not dealing directly with professional practice, significantly affected pharmacy. Revamped state drug (and food) laws remained in effect for intrastate control.

Books on the legal aspects of American pharmacy are essentially twentieth-century productions. However, the first publication in this category was a report on the status of legislation regulating the practice of pharmacy prepared by John M. Maisch in 1868. This report is presented here, together with five other pamphlets and books that illustrate the character, scope, variations, and definitions of the federal, state, and local laws of the late nineteenth and early twentieth centuries.

Proceedings, surveys, yearbooks, and reports of studies are valuable primary sources. Under "Other Books," nine titles illustrate this type of pharmaceutical literature, which deals with such topics as the general status of pharmacy practice, the education and research situations, economic aspects, and trends in the use and character of prescription drugs.

Pharmaceutical trade catalogs, the final category of the literature here considered, are valuable sources in their unique way for the economic, professional and technological history of pharmacy. Thirteen representative examples feature equipment, furniture, utensils, glassware, and drugstore sundries, in addition to crude drugs, galenicals, patent medicines, prescription specialties, and medicinal chemicals.

ACKNOWLEDGEMENTS

The preparation of this booklet and the microfiche editions it has stimulated should yield some sense of satisfaction to all those who cooperated with me so generously on one or the other facet of the project. I am particularly grateful to Professor Glenn Sonnedecker, whose idea it was, and who freely offered his time, knowledge, and concern. Others to whom I am indebted for skillful assistance include: the staff of the University of Wisconsin-Madison Libraries, particularly the historical section of the William S. Middleton Health Sciences Library, of the Rare Book Department and the Interlibrary Loan Department of the Memorial Library, and of the Frederick B. Power Pharmaceutical Library; the staff of the History of Medicine Division of the National Library of Medicine (Bethesda, Maryland); and the staff of the American Institute of the History of Pharmacy, particularly Elaine C. Stroud, Rosemary Zurlo-Cuva, and Gregory Higby. To the Institute I am grateful for the use of its resources in Madison, for some travel subsidy at one point in my investigations, and for publication of the booklet.

With appreciation I acknowledge the valuable suggestions made by David L. Cowen, Alex Berman, and John Parascandola, who critically reviewed the manuscript.

Finally, my sincere thanks to my close family and friends who helped to alleviate the strains of writing in a second language.— *NMK*

PART ONE: CATEGORICAL LIST OF SELECTED WORKS, WITH DESCRIPTIVE ESSAYS

A. DISPENSATORIES

A1 CULPEPER, Nicholas, 1616–1654

Pharmacopoeia Londinensis; or, the London dispensatory further adorned by the studies and collections of the fellows now living of the said college. Boston: John Allen, Printer, 1720. [24], 305 p., [35]. 11.5×18.5 cm. (Evans 2114) (DNLM) **AIHP 09**

Medical books in the American Colonies were of practical use not only for practitioners of medicine and pharmacy, but also for home treatment. Not surprisingly, the first medical book known to have been published in North America dealt with the preparation and use of medicines, and seems to have been a popular self-medication aid. This book was a reprint of Culpeper's English translation of the second (1650) edition of the *London Pharmacopoeia*. It is representative of early pharmaco-historical literature published in this country and illustrates the kinds and purposes of medicines of the time. Its professional impact has not been proven; but apparently it was commonly used in household medicine.

Published nearly seventy years after the initial translation (1653) already had gone through at least sixteen printings, this American 1720 edition omits or repeats parts of the original material. It exemplifies the transference of Galenic drug therapy to British North America, with a distinct turn towards domestic treatment of sickness. Arranged in two sections, the first part of the book includes compound preparations by classes—such as waters and tinctures—listed under their Latin names, with English names given as synonyms, and spells out the formulas and procedures for preparing medicaments. Culpeper's own critical comments, particularly regarding properties and uses, generally follow.

The second section of the book, a "Catalogue of Simples," classifies plant and animal drugs according to Galen (hot, cold, dry, moist), by the parts of the body they affected (e.g., head, neck, stomach, etc.), and by their properties (e.g., mollifying, purging, etc.). Unfamiliar simples such as butchers broom, dwarf elder, and cuc-

1

umers [*sic*] wild, are listed alphabetically together with familiar ones like artichokes, beets, marshmallow, and onions.

A key to the medical systems of Galen and Hippocrates (thirty-three chapters) includes topics such as cautions in using medicines, "what urine is," "what diuretics are," "of medicines easing pain," "cautions concerning purges," etc.

Nicholas Culpeper, an English physician who had been apprenticed to an apothecary, reputedly wrote a remarkable number of herbals and books on materia medica by the time of his death at age thirty-eight. His Puritanism, polemics and sometimes mystifying medical ideas permeated his works and made him a controversial figure.

A2 The Edinburgh new dispensatory. Containing I The Elements of pharmaceutical chemistry. II The Materia medica. III The Pharmaceutical and medicinal compositions of the new editions of the London (1788) and Edinburgh (1783) pharmacopoeias. Philadelphia: T. Dobson, Printer, 1791. 3 *l*, vii–xxii, 33–656 p. 12.5×20 cm. (Evans 23503) (WU) **AIHP 16**

This American edition of the *Edinburgh New Dispensatory*, the first of at least five editions published in the United States between 1791 and 1818, was reprinted from a British edition issued in 1789 by Andrew Duncan, Sr., a notable Edinburgh physician, later professor and president of the Royal College of Physicians. A comprehensive textbook of pharmacy having wide circulation in this country, it was the first book of consequence in the emergence of an American medico-pharmaceutical literature, particularly dispensatories.

Including all the pharmaceutical preparations of the London (1788) and Edinburgh (1783) pharmacopoeias, as well as formulas from other European pharmacopoeias, the book is divided into three parts. The first, Elements of Pharmacy (adapted to chemical principles), includes observations and explanations on the properties and relations of medicinal substances and on pharmaceutical apparatus and operations, illustrated with engravings. The second part, Materia Medica, contains mostly an account of the natural and medical history of medicinal substances, arranged alphabetically. The third part categorizes preparations by dosage forms—such as salts, spirits, powders, and pills—organized according to the London pharmacopoeia.

The preface eloquently reveals the stance on which this influential work was compiled: "We are indeed fully sensible, that in many particulars, with regard to the effects of medicines, and still more with regard to their mode of operation, even the best informed moderns are still in a state of ignorance and uncertainty. But we have at least endeavoured, as far as we are able, to shake off the trammels of theory and the authority of great names .... We are, however, very far from considering it as a complete system of practical and scientific pharmacy."

A3 THACHER, James, 1754–1844

The American new dispensatory. Containing general principles of pharmaceutic chemistry. Pharmaceutic operations. Chemical analysis of the articles of materia medica. Materia medica including several new and valuable articles, the production of the United States. Preparations and compositions .... Boston: T. B. Wait & Co., 1810. 3 *l*, 7–529 p. 13×20 cm. (Evans 21476) (WU) **AIHP 72**

Thacher's is the first clearly American creation of its kind: compiled by an American physician, based mainly on an American pharmacopoeia (the *Pharmacopoeia of the Massachusetts Medical Society*, see B2), and including articles of the native materia medica (drawn mainly from Barton's *Collections for an Essay*, see C14). Although Thacher acknowledged the influence of the *Edinburgh New Dispensatory*, his book reflected more of an American outlook than the *American Dispensatory* of John Redman Coxe (1806), which was based essentially on the authoritative Scottish work.

The *American New Dispensatory* (four editions through 1821) was used extensively in the early nineteenth century. Its purpose was to aid the practice of medical instructors and students by providing information more up-to-date than that in current analogous publications on the basics of pharmacy, pharmaceutical chemistry, and materia medica.

The text follows the nomenclature and arrangement of the *Massachusetts Pharmacopoeia*, hence of the ninth edition of the *Edinburgh Pharmacopoeia* (1803). In structure it has an introduction, (in which pharmacy and materia medica are defined), three parts, an appendix, and five tables. The first part contains general principles of pharmaceutical chemistry, pharmaceutical operations, and chemical analysis of the articles of the materia medica. In the second part (covering the materia medica), medicines are classified into twenty-one classes on the basis of function, and an overview of their operation on the living system is given. Both parts were adopted essentially from Murray's *Elements of Materia Medica and Pharmacy* (see C13). The third part features twenty-one categories

of preparations. The appendix includes topics such as medical prescriptions, the nature and medicinal uses of gases, and the method
of preparing American opium. The tables contain synonyms of ancient and systematic names; proportions of antimony, opium, and
quicksilver in some compound medicines; and posology.

The author, a Boston physician, had served in the Revolutionary Army, where he obtained wide experience in medicine and
surgery. Retiring from the army in 1783, he continued active medical practice and writing until his death at age ninety-one. Interested
in the development of botany for the uses of medicine, he was looked
upon as a good teacher of medicine. A prolific writer, *American
Medical Biography* (1828) is considered his principal work.

A4 WOOD, George B., 1797–1879 and BACHE, Franklin,
1792–1864

The dispensatory of the United States of America.
Philadelphia: Grigg & Elliot, 1833. 1 *l*, v–x,1 *l*, 1073 p.
15×21 cm. (WU) **AIHP 82**

About twelve years after the last edition of Thacher's *American
New Dispensatory* (see A3), physicians George B. Wood and Franklin Bache wrote this book as a needed commentary to the 1831
Philadelphia revision of the *Pharmacopoeia of the United States*
(see B4), of which they were the principal authors.

This first edition of the *United States Dispensatory* is a comprehensive source of information on what was then important in a
practical sense about pharmaceutical preparations and operations,
and on materia medica in the United States in the 1830s. No other
works of this kind relating exclusively to this country existed. It
represents the contemporary American state of the art.

The general division of medicines, the alphabetical arrangement, and the nomenclature follow the *Pharmacopoeia* of 1831.
However, the *United States Dispensatory* incorporates essential parts
of the pharmacopoeias of London, Edinburgh, and Dublin. Also, it
describes other medicinal substances of past or contemporary useful
reputation, and gives brief accounts of substances from other coun-
tries mentioned in the local medical literature.

The description of natural drugs includes information such as
natural history, place of growth or production, method of collection
and preparation for the market, commercial history, properties,
chemical composition and character, accidental or fraudulent adulteration, medical properties and applications, and pharmaceutical
processing. For a chemical preparation, the method and principles
of manufacture are given together with the other technicalities. For

botanical drugs, descriptions of indigenous and cultivated medicinal plants are given, as well as explanations of the toxicological effects of poisons, their antidotes, and detection by reagents.

The *United States Dispensatory* has gone through twenty-seven editions up to the present time. Until the twenty-fifth edition (1960), it was a comprehensive encyclopedic commentary on domestic and foreign drugs, including many historical references. Thereafter it concentrated more selectively on current information about pharmacologically effective medicines. For an example of an early twentieth century edition, see A6.

A similar book, though less influential and essentially medically oriented, competed temporarily with the *United States Dispensatory*. It was the *National Dispensatory*, published in five editions from 1879 to 1893. The first four editions were by physician Alfred Stillé and pharmacist John Maisch; the fifth by Stillé, Henry C. Maisch, and Charles Caspari, Jr.

The association between George B. Wood and Franklin Bache left a lasting influence on American pharmacy. Physician Wood was one of the most renowned teachers of his time, teaching chemistry and materia medica at the Philadelphia College of Pharmacy, and materia medica and theory and practice of medicine at the University of Pennsylvania. In his teaching, Wood pioneered the introduction of living specimens of medicinal plants, diagrams, charts, and models. He was a voluminous writer, president of the College of Physicians of Philadelphia and of the American Medical Association, and for several decades a determining force in the revision of the U.S. Pharmacopoeia.

Physician Bache practiced in Philadelphia after three years in the army. His interests included lecturing, writing, and scientific research. Bache was professor of chemistry at the Franklin Institute, the Philadelphia College of Pharmacy, and at the Jefferson Medical College, among other appointments. As a writer he contributed many worthwhile articles, and contributed extensively to the *American Cyclopedia of Medicine and Surgery*.

A5 KING, John, 1813–1893, and NEWTON, Robert S[afford], 1818–1881

The eclectic dispensatory of the United States of America. Authorized by the Eclectic National Medical Convention. Cincinnati: H. W. Derby & Co., 1852. 1 *l*, v–viii, 708 p. 14×21 cm. (WU) **AIHP 29**

The Eclectic Dispensatory of the United States is a landmark of the eclectic school of medical thought, a descendent of the botanico-medical movement of the first half of the nineteenth century whose impact was fully felt in pharmacy. It is a specialized formulary and commentary of "eclectic" drugs, not based on any pharmacopoeia, but similar to the usual English and American dispensatories.

The book presents all the substances recognized as medicinal by the Eclectic National Medical Convention, for the benefit of druggists and physicians. Except for a few instances, the nomenclature is that of the third revision of the *United States Pharmacopoeia*. In the first part the articles of the materia medica are arranged alphabetically under the Latin name of the plants from which they derive, giving the English names, botanical classification, history (description), properties, uses, and preparations. It includes remedial agents and preparations peculiar to eclectic practice and not found in any other contemporaneous medical work.

The second part includes officinal preparations* in alphabetical order by Latin names, followed by English names, preparations, properties, and uses. Here we also learn about the collection and preservation of plants and the composition of botanical drugs.

The appendix contains information in relation to weights and measures, abbreviations and Latin terms used in medicine, etc.

Many authoritative books and journals were consulted by the authors of the *Eclectic Dispensatory* and they were able to include considerable information not found in any other current American publication. The book underwent nineteen editions, mainly reprints, up to 1909, and three title changes: *The American Eclectic Dispensatory* (1854), *The American Dispensatory* (1859), and *King's American Dispensatory* (1898–1900).

Physicians John King and Robert S. Newton were professors at the Cincinnati Eclectic Medical Institute when they prepared this book, King in obstetrics and diseases of women and children, and Newton in surgery. Both had been teaching previously at the Memphis Institute.

Born in New York, John King was a pioneer eclectic expert on drugs, and graduate of the Beach Reformed Medical School directed by Wooster Beach. He was the discoverer of several plant constituents (e.g., podophyllin, macrotin) and introduced hydrastis and sanguinaria.

---

*Ambiguity surrounds the terms "officinal" and "official" as they were used in the nineteenth century. Originally used to designate preparations kept in the shop, the term "officinal" came to refer to preparations or substances that were included in a pharmacopoeia during the mid-nineteenth century. By the end of the century we find the following situation as characterized by Remington (*The Practice of Pharmacy*, third ed., 1894, p. 26, fn.1): "The word 'official' is now used to designate pharmacopoeial substances or preparations, the term 'officinal' being obsolete in this connection; the latter is properly applied to substances or preparations kept in the shop but not recognized by a pharmacopoeia."

Co-author Robert S. Newton, a native of Ohio and graduate of the University of Louisville, was well known as editor of the *Eclectic Medical Journal* from 1851 to 1861, and as an organizer of the National Eclectic Medical Association and the Eclectic Medical Society of New York.

A6 WOOD, Horatio C., Jr., 1874–1958 and LAWALL, Charles H., 1871–1937

The dispensatory of the United States of America. Twenty-first edition. Philadelphia and London: J.B. Lippincott Co., [c. 1926]. 3 *l*, iii–xxx, 1792 p. 17.5×25.5 cm. (WU)

The oldest commentary on drugs in continuous publication in the United States, the *United States Dispensatory* (see A4 for first edition) has remained a remarkably popular reference book in this country and, in some degree, overseas. The twenty-first edition, published nearly 100 years after the first edition, still retains an encyclopedic character. It is listed here as a representative of this type of literature in the late 1920s and as a useful source for the history of drugs then in use. The many literature references, a distinctive feature of past editions, are substantially augmented in this edition, "not only to give the sources of the most recent studies . . . but also to furnish . . . the key which will unlock the door of the past to those who may wish to trace the history of the development of some phase of the subject."

After an introductory segment—including the preface, an explanatory note, a list of abbreviations, The Food and Drug Act and the Harrison Narcotic Act—the text is divided into three parts. Part I includes all the drugs and preparations of the *United States Pharmacopoeia* (1926) and the *British Pharmacopoeia* (1914), and the crude drugs of the *National Formulary* (1926), arranged in alphabetical sequence by their Latin titles. For each substance the monograph includes the official title and definition, unofficial synonyms, sources and history, description and physical properties, assay method, adulterants, chemical constituents, incompatibilities, therapeutic uses, toxicology, dosage, and a list of preparations.

Part II covers unofficial drugs (drugs not included in the legal standards), particularly new remedies, arranged alphabetically by English names.

Part III contains general tests, processes and apparatus, reagents, test solutions and tables of U.S.P. X; and of the *British Pharmacopoeia* (1914), a summary of the galenical preparations of the 1926 *National Formulary* (1926); and formulas for reagents used in clinical examinations.

Physician and pharmacologist Horatio Charles Wood, Jr., and pharmacist and chemist Charles Herbert LaWall were colleagues in the Philadelphia College of Pharmacy when they edited this edition of the *United States Dispensatory*, with the assistance of pharmacists Heber W. Youngken and Ivor Griffith, and physician John F. Anderson.

Born in Philadelphia, Wood was a nephew of George B. Wood, one of the editors of the first fourteen editions of the book (1833–1879). He received an M.D. degree from the University of Pennsylvania in 1896, followed by research work in Bern and Turin during the next two years. His academic career of about fifty years included appointments at the University of Pennsylvania (demonstrator in pharmaco-dynamics, 1898–1907, and professor of pharmacology and therapeutics, 1916–1942), the Medico-Chirurgical College of Philadelphia (professor of pharmacology and therapeutics, 1910–1916), and in the Philadelphia College of Pharmacy and Science (professor of pharmacology, 1921–1950). He was a member of the Committee of Revision of the *Pharmacopoeia* for three decades (1910–1940) and vice president of the Pharmacopoeial Convention in 1941. He was co-editor of four editions of the *United States Dispensatory* (twentieth, 1918, through twenty-third, 1948) and author of *A Textbook of Pharmacology* (1912).

Charles LaWall was a native of Allentown, Pennsylvania, and graduated from the Philadelphia College of Pharmacy (Ph.G., 1893 and Ph.M., 1905). He received an Sc.D. from Susquehanna University (1920) and an honorary Pharm.D. degree from the University of Pittsburgh in 1919. Active in community pharmacy, the pharmaceutical industry, education, and government, his professional involvement extended over forty years including membership on the revision committees of the U.S. Pharmacopoeia and National Formulary. He was president of both the American Pharmaceutical Association (1919), and the American Association of Colleges of Pharmacy (1923). A prolific author, his *Four Thousand Years of Pharmacy* (1927) was the first history of pharmacy book written by an American and published in this country. In 1928 he received the Remington Medal for distinguished work in pharmacy.

B. PHARMACOPOEIAS AND FORMULARIES

B1 [BROWN, William], 1748–1792

Pharmacopoeia simpliciorum et efficaciorum in usum nosocomii militaris. Philadelphia: Styner & Cist., 1778. 4–32 p. 9.5×16 cm. (Evans 15750) (DNLM) **AIHP 06**

Widely known as the "Lititz Pharmacopoeia," this work marks the beginning of an American pharmaceutical formulary tradition. Apparently the first publication on American soil to be termed a pharmacopoeia, it is historically noteworthy as the first attempt to standardize the compounding and dispensing of medicines in the United States albeit within the military establishment. In addition, it contains the first authoritative allusion to large-scale preparation of medicines in this country, and implies for the first time that the compounder and dispenser of medicines must have some knowledge and skills in pharmaceutical techniques, thus recognizing the importance of the task.

Although the booklet bore the title "Pharmacopoeia," it was just a small emergency formulary—not a pharmacopoeia in the modern sense—published during the Revolutionary War, for the use of the military hospitals set up in Lititz and in Bethlehem. About half of the formulas were from the author's experience and that of his American colleagues, the rest mostly from the *Edinburgh Pharmacopoeia* (1756), but other European sources were also used. It is divided into two parts: one presents formulas for eighty-four internal remedies, such as waters, electuaries, pills, powders, tinctures, syrups, fomentations, gargarisms, conserves, mucilages, and other dosage forms, and frequently gives therapeutic indications and dosages. The other part lists sixteen surgical medicaments, mostly plasters and ointments for external use.

Written in Latin, this hospital formulary gives directions for the preparation of medicines, or refers the user to the Edinburgh or London pharmacopoeias. These details suggest that it was intended for the trained apothecary or physician. Adapted for use in the field, this formulary is brief because not many drugs were on hand. It includes "universal potions," like barley, rice, and toasted bread waters to be alternated as necessary; it permits substitution, such as linseed oil for olive oil, and cider for vinegar, and the interchange of plant parts, such as roots, bark or wood; and it includes indigenous drugs such as sassafras and serpentaria. Issuance of a reprint three years later (1781) may indicate that it was found useful.

Although the first edition of this work was published anonymously, the circumstantial evidence suggests that William Brown, Physician General of the Middle Department of the Continental Army, probably was a principal author. At any rate, his name appears on the titlepage of the second edition (1781) as the presumptive author. Dr. Brown, a Scot, was a graduate of the University of Edinburgh (1770). In 1780 he resigned from his medical role in the Revolution to resume private practice. He was known as a skillful and diligent physician.

The "Lititz pharmacopoeia" brings to mind the second hospital formulary issued in this country, one designed for the relatively small French army fighting on the side of the American patriots:

Jean François Coste's *Compendium pharmaceuticum* (Newport, Rhode Island, 1780). This one however, being European in most respects, did not achieve the practical or historical significance of the former.

B2   The pharmacopoeia of the Massachusetts Medical Society. Boston: E. & J. Larkin, 1808. 3 *l*, v–x, 2 *l*, 3–272 p. 10×18 cm. (Evans 15554) (WU) **AIHP 56**

This book is a milestone in the development of drug reference standards in the United States, being the first of its nature issued by an organized medical group and for general civilian use—not just for the hospital military, like the earlier "Lititz pharmacopoeia" (see B1).

Significantly, the preface recognizes the American apothecary as a distinctive compounder of medicines, *vis à vis* the physician as a prescriber. With only the authority of the Massachusetts Medical Society behind it, it was not a pharmacopoeia legally obligatory in the modern sense, but was a manual to enhance communication between physicians and apothecaries by establishing uniform pharmaceutical preparations and nomenclature, a manual to "be handled by those, who are well versed in chemistry, well acquainted with the characters of medicinal substances, and familiarly accustomed to pharmaceutical operations."

Based primarily on the influential *Edinburgh Pharmacopoeia* (Ninth Edition, 1803), with the omissions, alterations and additions deemed necessary locally, it generally adopted the scientific botanical and chemical nomenclature of that standard. On the other hand, it includes some native drugs and, although Latin names with their English translations are used, directions are in English only.

The work lists about 536 drugs and preparations as well as the best methods of preparation. It is organized in two parts with a section of tables. Part I lists about 250 articles of the materia medica in alphabetical order by Latin names, including the English names and the parts used or descriptions of the articles. In twenty-one chapters, corresponding to classes of preparations, Part II contains the Latin and English names, formulas, and procedures of about 280 drug products. Finally, each of four tables gives, respectively, the proportion of antimony, opium and quicksilver in some compound medicines; doses of drugs and correct pronunciation of their names; ancient names; and systematic names.

This pharmacopoeia was the foundation of the first unmistakably American dispensatory: Thacher's *American New Dispensatory*, 1810 (see A3). In addition, more than ninety percent of an unpublished revision was later included in the first edition of the *Pharmacopoeia of the United States*, 1820 (see B4). Reflecting the modernization of the contemporaneous *Edinburgh Pharmacopoeia*, the *Pharmacopoeia of the Massachusetts Medical Society* is an important primary source on early nineteenth-century drug therapy and technology.

B3 Pharmacopoeia nosocomii Neo-Eboracensis; or the pharmacopoeia of the New York Hospital ... an appendix containing a general posological table and a comparative view of the former and present terms in materia medica and pharmacy. New York: Collins & Co., 1816. 2 *l*, vi–x, 1 *l*, 180, 1 p. 12×20 cm. (Evans 38453) (WU) **AIHP 57**

The New York Hospital, the second hospital of its kind in the United States (founded 1771), was the source of one of the earliest records of hospital pharmacy in this country and of the first two civilian hospital formularies. The first civilian hospital formulary, authored by the physician Valentine Seaman, was the *Pharmacoepia [sic] Chirurgica* of 1811, a little manual without any institutional authority or discernible influence. The second one, the formulary introduced here, represented a fresh start five years after Seaman's initial effort, and was co-authored by him and Samuel L. Mitchill, a leader in the subsequent issuance of the *United States Pharmacopoeia* (see B4). It bore the authority of the physicians and surgeons of the hospital and is looked upon as the beginning of this type of pharmaceutical literature in the U.S.A.

The *Pharmacopoeia of the New York Hospital*, a pharmacopoeia only in the original meaning of "to make remedies," is historically noteworthy as the first precedent-setting attempt to systematize the preparing of medicines in a hospital starting from the prescribing views and opinions of the medical staff. Issued principally for the hospital apothecary and the medical students, one of its declared purposes was "effecting reform in the pharmaceutical department," but it was envisioned that it could be useful to other apothecaries not having a "regular Pharmacopoeia" on hand.

This work lists about 170 simples and around 260 preparations in alphabetical sequence by Latin titles, formulas selected from one of the pharmacopoeias of Great Britain, extemporaneous prescriptions suggested by the hospital physicians and surgeons, and some native products not found in the existing treatises on materia medica and pharmacy. It also includes the weights and measures adopted in the hospital, explanations and abbreviations of terms frequently used in prescriptions, directions for collecting and preserving medicinal vegetables, the diet table of the hospital, synonyms of the simples and preparations, and doses.

B4   The pharmacopoeia of the United States of America. By the authority of the Medical Societies and Colleges. Boston: Wells and Lilly, Printers, Dec. 1820. 2 *l*, 5–272 p. 12×18 cm. (AIHP) **AIHP 58**

As a prelude to the legal standardization of medicines in the United States, the appearance of this volume was a notable pharmaco-historic event. By selecting a materia medica and corresponding preparations and compounds, and establishing a convenient and definite nomenclature, adhering to the best state of current medical and pharmaceutical knowledge, it inaugurated a trend that persists today.

Published by authority of the medical profession, various sources were used in its compilation, among them most of a complete unpublished revision of the *Pharmacopoeia of the Massachusetts Medical Society*, which itself was based primarily on the *Edinburgh Pharmacopoeia* (see B2).

The scope of this book of standards revolved around the admittance of drugs "the utility of which is most fully established and understood" and of "native articles . . . which were considered to possess qualities sufficiently important, or which were found to be much employed by practitioners." However, substances "the claims of which are of a more uncertain kind" were also included, but on a secondary list.

The section on preparations and compositions includes, in alphabetical order, only formulas recognized by American or European physicians and expected to be prepared by the practitioners of pharmacy themselves. Officinal compounds not necessarily to be prepared by the individual practitioner, are listed in the section on materia medica; thus the large-scale manufacture of medicines is again implied in a work of this kind (see B1). The entire work is written in English, but the nomenclature and all essential parts are also in Latin.

Physicians Lyman Spalding and Samuel L. Mitchill were the principal forces behind this work: Mitchill providing incentive and support and Spalding executing a plan based on democratic representation. Jacob Bigelow, a well-known physician and botanist, member of the Pharmacopoeial Convention, and author of the botanical part of the book, independently prepared a supplemental volume explaining the origin, qualities, medical uses, and modes of prescription and administration of the simples and compounds included in the *Pharmacopoeia (A Treatise of Materia Medica*, 1822).

In addition to a slightly modified version of the first edition published in Boston in 1828, two second editions were issued—one in New York in 1830 and the other in Philadelphia in 1831. The former was of little consequence, but the latter came to be accepted as U.S.P. I (i.e., First Revision) and was the progenitor of successive revisions. Other landmark editions are U.S.P. VI (see B7) and U.S.P. VIII (see B14).

B5   GRIFFITH, R. Eglesfeld, 1798–1850

A universal formulary: containing the methods of preparing and administering officinal and other medicines. The whole adapted to physicians and pharmaceutists. Philadelphia: Lea and Blanchard, 1850. 2 *l*, viii–ix, 9–567 p. 14.5×22.5 cm. (DNLM) **AIHP 21**

Books of formulas were popular among practitioners of pharmacy for the preparation of medicines in nineteenth-century America, some preceding the founding of the *United States Pharmacopoeia*, and others appearing after the founding of the *National Formulary*. Compiled by individual or collective authors, and having diverse objectives and contents, these unpretentious manuals were intended to fulfill most of the needs of the ordinary compounder and dispenser of medicines.

The formulary represented here is one of the earliest by an individual author. It contains a concise collection of formulas, pharmaceutical processes, and other general practical information for physicians and pharmacists. Its sources were many, but the author cites particularly the *United States Pharmacopoeia* (1842), the Mohr-Redwood-Procter *Practical Pharmacy* (1849) (see C1), and his own *Medical Botany* (1847) (see C20). William Procter, Jr., included this formulary in his 1856 list of reference works recommended to pharmacists.

An extensive introduction covers topics such as weights and measures, specific gravity, temperatures for certain pharmaceutical operations, prescribing vocabulary, observations on the management of the sickroom, doses and rules for the administration of medicines, and management of convalescence and relapses. This is followed by about 300 pages of formulas arranged alphabetically, indicating the source of each formula. The names and the quantities of the ingredients are spelled out in English, not abbreviated as was customary. Next are some dietetic formulas not included with the others, a list of incompatibles, a table of doses of the most important medicines, a table of pharmaceutical names which differ in the United States and the British pharmacopoeias, concise observations and directions on officinal preparations taken mostly from Mohr-Redwood-Procter's *Practical Pharmacy*, a brief survey of poisons and their antidotes, an index of diseases and their remedies, an index of pharmaceutical and botanical names, and a general index.

This formulary went through several editions, of which the third (1874) was revised and enlarged by John M. Maisch.

A native of Philadelphia, Robert Eglesfeld Griffith had graduated in medicine from the University of Pennsylvania in 1820. An assiduous student, he became interested in many branches of science and was a pioneer in American pharmacognosy. Among his positions, he served as editor of the *Journal of the Philadelphia College of Pharmacy* (later titled *American Journal of Pharmacy*) from 1831–1836, physician to the Board of Health in Philadelphia (1833–1836), professor of materia medica at the Philadelphia College of Pharmacy for a year (1835), then professor of materia medica, therapeutics, hygiene, and medical jurisprudence at the University of Maryland. In 1838 he was professor of obstetrics and medical jurisprudence at the University of Virginia, returning to practice in Philadelphia in 1839. Among other books, he authored *Chemistry for the Four Seasons* (1846) and *Medical Botany* (1847) (see C20).

B6 KILNER, Walter B., b. 1847

A compendium of modern pharmacy and druggists' formulary. Containing the recent methods of manufacturing and preparing elixirs, tinctures, fluid extracts, flavoring extracts, emulsions, perfumery and toilet articles, wines and liquors; also physician's prescriptions, liniments, pills, powders, ointments, syrups, antidotes to poisons, weights and measures, and miscellaneous information indispensible to the pharmacist. Springfield, IL: H.W. Rokker, Printer, 1880. 1 *l*, 3–478 p. 13.5×18.5 cm. (DNLM) **AIHP 28**

A compilation of tested and approved formulas "gathered from an astonishingly large number of volumes, all of which no man's private library would be likely to contain," and from "eminently successful pharmaceutical chemists," Kilner's formulary is a suitable representation of "elegant preparations" as they were in the 1880s. As a reference guide for druggists and pharmacists, it offered a comprehensive—but compact and handy—formulary containing only formulas, except for brief observations on weights and measures.

In thirty-two chapters, the *Compendium* gives the latest contemporary methods for making tinctures, fluid extracts, flavoring extracts, specific medications, essences, elixirs, solutions, syrups, infusions, medicated waters, emulsions, physicians' prescriptions, liniments, pills, medicated wines, powders, ointments, miscellaneous preparations, perfumery and toilet articles, and others. Each chapter covers one class of preparations, the formulas being arranged alphabetically by Latin names and numbered in sequence.

Enlarged editions containing other information besides formulas were published for at least fifteen years. Another formulary published concurrently with the later editions was *Fenner's Working Formulae* (Byron Fenner, Westfield, NY, 1884), which merits mention here because it was so widely known. However, Fenner's book was different in scope, being essentially a comparison of the 1870 and 1880 revisions of the *Pharmacopoeia of the United States*, with the addition of some methods claimed to be superior to the official ones.

Born in England, Walter B. Kilner went to Indiana as a boy with his father, a physician. Later they moved to Illinois. At age eighteen he opened a drugstore with his brother (1865), and practiced pharmacy in Illinois for many years.

B7 The pharmacopoeia of the United States of America. Sixth decennial revision. By authority of the National Convention for Revising the Pharmacopoeia held at Washington, A.D. 1880. New York: William Wood & Co., 1882. xli, 487 p. 14×22 cm. (WU) **AIHP 59**

This is one of the most significant pieces of American pharmaceutical literature, not only for ushering in the modern pattern of the Pharmacopoeia, but also for its part in the subsequent improvement of drug standards in this country. The changed format, with the monographs arranged alphabetically and fully described and explained, and the perception of the community pharmacist more as an overseer of the quality than as a preparer of medicines, had far-reaching effects on future revisions.

The most significant innovations of U.S.P. VI include: tests of purity for many chemicals, with limits for unavoidable impurities and fixed tests for the absence of adulterants; assays of some drugs, including alkaloids; more substantial description of the physical characteristics of vegetable and mineral simples, and where possible, the introduction of chemical properties, formulas and molecular weights; more emphasis on the directions for keeping and preserving crude drugs, chemicals, and preparations; and the listing at the end of each monograph for a basic, active drug its various official dosage forms.

Of 997 monographs, 256 were additions, while 229 titles were deleted from the previous edition. Several classes of preparations were significantly reduced, such as decoctions and infusions, and suppositories were eliminated altogether. Abstracts were introduced as a dosage form, and more fluid extracts, syrups, and tinctures were included.

This precedent-setting drug reference standard was prepared by a Committee of Revision presided over by a learned hospital pharmacist, Charles Rice of Bellevue Hospital, New York, a central figure in upgrading the pharmacopoeia. A majority of the Committee members were pharmacists, among them Oscar Oldberg and Otto A. Wall who subsequently co-authored a commentary and supplement titled *A Companion to the United States Pharmacopoeia* (New York, 1884). It was a voluminous reference book and working manual for pharmacists, physicians and students, reminiscent of the *Companion to the British Pharmacopoeia*. Only two editions were published. Following earlier European models, American booklets (whether termed epitome, conspectus, or pocket guide) also appeared, extracting official drug compendia to provide the essentials most often needed by prescribing physicians.

B8 The national formulary of unofficinal preparations. By authority of the American Pharmaceutical Association. n.p.: American Pharmaceutical Association, 1888. ix, 176 p. 15×21 cm. (WU) **AIHP 41**

This first edition is historically noteworthy as the starting point of what became one of the two important legal standards for drugs in the United States. Other formularies and the noted U.S.P. VI (see B7) were in use at the time of its publication. But the deletion of many formulas from the Pharmacopoeia that were still valued by practitioners, the diversity of unofficinal formularies, and the manufacture and persistent prescribing of formulas as brand products were motivating forces behind its issuance. Intended for pharmacists and physicians, it was hoped that physicians would prescribe "preparations made in accordance with the formulae contained therein, instead of designating any special maker's product."

This formulary was put together by a Committee of the American Pharmaceutical Association chaired by the well-known hospital pharmacist Charles Rice, who was simultaneously chairman of the Committee of Revision of the *United States Pharmacopoeia*, and had presided over the issuance of the remarkable Sixth Revision.

The *National Formulary* was founded on the principle of frequency of use, mainly as an unofficial supplement to the *Pharmacopoeia*. It presented 435 formulas arranged alphabetically and numbered in sequence, gathered from existing formularies or contributed by individuals or groups. Two interesting features are (1) formulas "constructed on rational principles ... mainly with regard to uniform composition and reliable effect," as substitutes for some popular nostrums, and (2) the listing of thirteen "basic preparations" from which most of the formulas could be prepared.

The third edition of the *National Formulary* (N.F. III, 1905), was given legal authority like the U.S.P. VIII (see B14) by virtue of the 1906 Federal Food and Drug Act. In consequence, the next edition appeared under the abridged title the *National Formulary* (dropping the term "unofficinal"). Initially different from the *United States Pharmacopoeia* in scope and purpose, the *National Formulary* eventually became analogous to it, which, with other considerations, led to the consolidation of the two standards (U.S.P. XXI-N.F. XVI, 1985).

B9 OLESON, Charles W[ilmot], 1842–1906

Secret nostrums and systems of medicine. A book of formulas. Chicago: Oleson & Co., 1890. 1 *l*, 3–206 p. 12×17.5 cm. (DNLM) **AIHP 45**

American medical and pharmaceutical periodicals of the late nineteenth and early twentieth centuries often published formulas which they claimed were identical (or nearly identical) to those of popular nostrums. These formulas usually were obtained either through access to specific secret recipes or through experimental approximation. The book presented here collects more than 340 of these formulas, as published in over twenty journals and related publications. A few non-proprietary formulas and some secret methods or systems of treatment are also included.

A large number of the formulas came from the laboratories of Frederick Stearns & Co., Detroit, and were published originally in *New Idea*, a house organ that regularly inveighed against secrecy of composition of drug products. Other formulas appeared in such journals as *Medical World* (Philadelphia) and *Western Druggist* (Chicago). Among the contributors were well-known chemists such as F. Hoffmann (see C37), Albert Prescott, and A. B. Lyons (see C38).

The formulas appear alphabetically under the names of the medicaments, and are accompanied by physical descriptions and preparation procedures, and the sources of each formula. Critical annotations of a large number of the formulas include remarks on uses, claimed effectiveness, poisonous nature, and recommendations for or against their use. In a few cases just the composition without quantities is given.

Examples of the nostrums represented in this book are Lydia Pinkham's Compound, Eno's Fruit Salt, Brown's Iron Bitters, Cleary's Asthma Powder, and Murray's Systemic Tonic.

Ten editions were published from 1890 to 1903.

Born in Portland, Maine, Charles Wilmot Oleson was a graduate of the Harvard Medical School (1866) who served in the Fourteenth Infantry during the Civil War. Oleson was licensed in Illinois, lived in Lombard until his death, and was a member of the Chicago Medical Society.

B10 EBERT, Albert E., 1840–1906 and HISS, A. Emil, b. 1866

> The standard formulary. A collection of over four thousand formulas for pharmaceutical preparations, family remedies, toilet articles, and miscellaneous preparations especially adapted to the requirements of retail druggists. Chicago: G.P. Engelhard & Co., 1896. 4 *l*, [11], 500 p. 15×22.5 cm. (WU) **AIHP 15**

This formulary presents a broad assortment of the most reliable unofficinal domestic and European product formulas available to American pharmacists at the end of the nineteenth century. Some of the formulas were collected from years of practical experience, including sources such as Edward Parrish's *An Introduction to Practical Pharmacy*, the *Eclectic Dispensatory*, and the *National Formulary*. Other formulas were selected from European authorities including the German manuals by Karl Dieterich and Hermann Hager, and the British, German, French, Swedish, Norwegian, Belgian, Austrian, and Italian pharmacopoeias.

Of its seven parts, Part I of the *Standard Formulary* is the most extensive, including about sixty types of pharmaceutical preparations, such as confections, glycerites, snuffs, Thompsonian [*sic*] remedies, and medicinal wines. Parts II to VI cover household remedies, proprietary preparations, veterinary preparations, toilet preparations, and soda water preparations. Part VII contains miscellaneous preparations. The formulas are arranged alphabetically by English names under type of preparation.

Revised and enlarged editions were published during the next twenty years or so, growing into a multi-volume work entitled *The New Standard Formulary* (1908).

Albert E. Ebert was born in Germany and A. Emil Hiss in France, with an age difference of twenty-six years between them. Both had settled in Chicago with their parents at an early age. Ebert acquired national fame in pharmacy for his many valuable contributions. He began his studies at the Chicago College of Pharmacy in 1859, and graduated from the Philadelphia College of Pharmacy in 1864. His quest for pharmaceutical knowledge took him to the University of Munich where he earned a Ph.D. degree in 1867. The following year Ebert opened a retail pharmacy in Chicago and began teaching at the College of Pharmacy. Active in the American Pharmaceutical Association, he served as its president in 1872, and established the Ebert Prize Fund for the stimulation of original pharmaceutical research. Other activities included membership in the Committee of Revision of the United States Pharmacopoeia for several decades, and on the State Board of Pharmacy of Illinois for five years.

The much younger Hiss matriculated in the Chicago College of Pharmacy in 1885 and received a Ph.G. degree in 1887. He served as an instructor of materia medica at the College and as professor of chemistry at the Chicago Veterinary College. Above all, he devoted himself to retail pharmacy, making several practical contributions to the pharmaceutical literature.

B11 Pharmacopoeia of the American Institute of Homoeopathy. Published for the Committee on Pharmacopoeia of the American Institute of Homoeopathy. Boston: Otis Clapp and Son, Agents, 1897. 2 *l*, 7–674 p. 15.5×22.5 cm. (WU) **AIHP 54**

Issued by the authority of the American Institute of Homoeopathy, this publication is historically interesting as the first edition of the only legalized drug standard in the United States pertaining to a medical sect. In preparation for at least nine years, the book was directed at physicians, pharmacists, students and instructors for the purpose of "diffusing useful knowledge, and promoting uniformity in the strength and quality of medicinal preparations and in their literature as well." Significantly, its introduction calls for instruction in the principles and practice of pharmacy in every medical college, adding that "pharmaceutical knowledge seems to be even more important to homoeopathic than to allopathic practitioners, for the reason that only a portion of the former are within easy reach of the professional pharmacist who understands the preparation of medicines for homoeopathic use."

Based mainly on the *British Homoeopathic Pharmacopoeia*, the book begins with about twenty pages of prefatory and introductory material, followed by three parts: Part I, on general pharmacy, deals with units of medicinal strength, utensils, menstrua, vehicles, prescriptions, etc.; Part II, special pharmaceutics, lists the drugs in alphabetical order by Latin names, followed by English names, natural order, synonyms in Latin and English, description, habitat, history, parts used and methods of preparation; Part III contains tables of abbreviations used in prescription writing, and of weights and measures, and atomic weights, plus a pronunciation guide.

From the third to the most recent eighth edition (1974) the book appeared under the title *Homoeopathic Pharmacopoeia of the United States*. Beginning with the fifth edition, it was recognized as an official compendium of drug standards by the Federal Food, Drug and Cosmetic Act of 1938.

Of earlier homeopathic pharmacopoeias without official status, the best known was the comparable *The American Homoeopathic Pharmacopoeia* published by F. E. Boericke and A. J. Tafel of Philadelphia in 1882. Boericke was later appointed to the twelve-member committee for the Institute's *Pharmacopoeia*, but reportedly he declined to serve.

B12 HISS, A. Emil, b. 1866

Thesaurus of proprietary preparations and pharmaceutical specialties. Including "patent" medicines, proprietary pharmaceuticals, open-formula specialties, synthetic remedies, etc. Chicago: G.P. Englehard & Co., 1899. 1 *l*, 4–279 p. 15×22.5 cm. (AIHP) **AIHP 24**

Published in 1898 and reprinted in 1899 and 1900, this book is in a class by itself: a formulary "not for duplicating the various preparations, but to give physicians and pharmacists an approximate idea of their composition and properties." Aiming to include all preparations not found in the contemporary *United States Pharmacopoeia*, dispensatories or other authoritative reference works, the *Thesaurus* is an extraordinary source of information on the composition and therapeutic properties of patent medicines, proprietary pharmaceuticals, open-formula specialties (non-proprietary pharmaceutical specialties), and synthetic remedies. Typical formulas representing thousands of proprietary formulations appear under class titles (as in "Balsams," "Cures," "Pills") or under therapeutic properties or claims (as in "Asthma Cures," "Rheumatism Remedies"). Formulas were reproduced freely from the *Standard Formulary* (Ebert and Hiss, 1896; see B10).

Compiled from product information supplied by numerous manufacturers, or from other sources, such as analyses and "clever guessing," the book was intended as a handy reference. It is arranged in a single alphabetical sequence, with listing either by dosage form or by therapeutic indication in two-column pages. In addition to the sources, descriptions, and applications for specific products, formulas and instructions for preparing similar preparations are included.

For a brief biographical sketch of the author see B10.

B13 The pharmacopoeia of the German Hospital of the city of Philadelphia. Including formulas for all stock preparations and the average doses of all drugs, chemicals, and preparations usually dispensed at the German Hospital pharmacy. Philadelphia: Board of Trustees, 1902. 1 *l*, 3–144 p. 8.5×16.5 cm. (WU) **AIHP 55**

This pocket-size hospital formulary follows in a long tradition of similar pharmaceutical manuals that were popular before the functional reassessment of the late 1920s. Its stated purpose was to give hospital physicians "a more accurate knowledge of the resources and contents of the Hospital Pharmacy."

After a brief preface, the main part of the formulary consists of an alphabetical list of drugs by English or Latin names, including English and Latin synonyms, minimum and maximum doses, preparations and, in some instances, formulas. Products of the *United States Pharmacopoeia* were given precedence, but many of the newest synthetic medicinals of the times, and a large number of substitute formulas for the more popular proprietaries were also included. Other sections consist of general directions in cases of poisoning, poisons and their antidotes, drugs classified according to their physiological action, maximum doses of potent drugs, comparative temperatures and comparative scales of weights and measures.

B14 The pharmacopoeia of the United States of America. Eighth decennial revision. By authority of the United States Pharmacopoeial Convention held at Washington, A.D. 1900. Official from September 1st 1905. Philadelphia: P. Blakiston's Son & Co. *l*, xxv, 692 p. 14×21 cm. (WU) **AIHP 60**

The first revision issued by the newly incorporated United States Pharmacopoeial Convention marked a new phase in the evolution of the *United States Pharmacopoeia*. The establishment of the corporation gave the *United States Pharmacopoeia* an enduring foundation; its legal recognition as a compendium of drug standards by the 1906 Pure Food and Drugs Act gave it a significant new social meaning since it had acquired the force of law. It became necessary to issue a modified printing of this eighth decennial revision of the *United States Pharmacopoeia*, and it was dated the year it took effect instead of the year of the Convention, as had been customary.

Besides the organizational changes taking effect with this revision, many technical improvements were introduced reflecting the pharmaceutical nature of quality assurances, with medical input "restricted mainly to deciding upon the admission or exclusion of articles." The innovative features of U.S.P. VIII include: use of the term "official" for substances and preparations recognized in it, a more accurate definition of the limit of purity by standards or rubrics of purity, assay processes for about twenty drugs and preparations, average approximate adult doses (instead of a minimum and a maximum) in the metric system, a small number of proprietary drugs and patented products of known composition and method of preparation, structural formulas for chemical compounds (in addition to empirical formulas), fewer synonyms in the text to discourage their use, adoption, in general, of a uniform strength of ten percent for tinctures of potent drugs, as recommended by the International Conference on the Unification of Potent Medicaments (1902), use of weights for solids, and measures for liquids, in the metric system, and the first biological (Antidiphtheric Serum) and glandular (thyroid and suprarenal) products.

Of 958 monographs (thirty-five less than in U.S.P. VII), 117 were additions, 151 titles having been deleted from the previous edition. However, more test and volumetric solutions and volumetric and gravimetric assays were included. An eighty-page appendix and fifteen tables supplement the text.

This landmark revision of the *United States Pharmacopoeia* was issued by a Committee of Revision in which eighteen of its twenty-five members were well-known pharmacists, including its prominent chairman, Joseph P. Remington. Moreover, for the next five decades the *United States Pharmacopoeia* exerted a discernible influence in Latin America through translation into the Spanish language.

B15 The druggists circular formula book. In which may be found recipes for hundreds of unofficial preparations in daily demand in the drugstore, the laboratory, the boudoir, the household . . .; together with a compilation of process outlines, notes, hints and other valuable information and suggestions for retail druggists and dispensing pharmacists culled from the pages of that publication. New York: The Druggists Circular, 1915. 2 *l*, 5–242 p. 15×21 cm. (WU) **AIHP 11**

This popular formula book brings together "some of the valuable information for druggists contained in the annual volumes of *The Druggists Circular*," which was the first American independent pharmacy journal of national circulation. In response to inquiries, this information was derived from a large number of books on pharmacy and the related arts and sciences, as well as formularies, leading medical and pharmaceutical journals, association proceedings, national and state bulletins, and similar publications.

Resembling some previous formularies in format and general purpose (e.g., B10), this volume contains recipes for hundreds of unofficial preparations frequently called for early in the century, as well as other useful information of pharmaceutical interest. The formulas include preparations for diverse technical uses. The composition of some nostrums is provided in brief abstract form, culled from reports of the food and drug departments of Connecticut, Ohio, Indiana, North Dakota, and New Hampshire, and from publications of American and British medical associations.

Intended as an immediate reference, the two-column text is illustrated with line drawings and indexed. In no specific order, the rubrics include descriptions or general information, instructions for use, formulas, and related compounds.

A second edition appeared in 1920, and the title was changed to *2896 Formulas for Pharmacists* in 1928. Shortly after, the book was superseded by another more comprehensive formulary, *The Pharmaceutical Recipe Book* (see B16).

B16 The pharmaceutical recipe book. By authority of the American Pharmaceutical Association. n.p.: The American Pharmaceutical Association, 1929. iii–vii, 454 p. 15×22.5 cm. (WU) **AIHP 52**

A collection of over 1000 commonly needed formulas, this book (in three editions) was widely used by American pharmacists during the 1930s and 1940s. The American Pharmaceutical Association compiled this reference work as a service to pharmacists after *The National Formulary* became a legal standard (see B8). The first edition of the *Pharmaceutical Recipe Book* was published following the third (1928) edition of the similar, but less comprehensive, *Druggist's Circular Formula Book* (see B15). Compilation of the formulas began as early as 1912, and over a five-year period beginning in 1916, more than 500 of them were serialized as a special section of the *Journal* of the Association.

Including only formulas considered "reliable and worthy" and excluding proprietary or trademark products, the book is divided into nine parts: Pharmaceutical Formulas, Hospital Formulas, Dental Formulas, Laboratory Reagents, Veterinary Formulas, Photographic Formulas, Cosmetic Formulas, Flavoring Extracts, and Technical and Miscellaneous Formulas. The contents of each part are arranged in alphabetical sequence under English titles, with Latin titles sometimes given as synonyms. Using mainly the metric system, each formula has working directions and special comments when necessary. Disclaiming any authority on the therapeutic value of the preparations, the doses are based on generally accepted practice.

Under the leadership of the prominent New York pharmacist J. Leon Lascoff (1867–1943) as Chairman of the Committee on the Recipe Book and the equally distinguished pharmacist-educator from Philadelphia, Ivor Griffith (1891–1961), as Editor, many well-known practitioners collaborated in the preparation of this book, including E. Fullerton Cook, Bernard Fantus, Robert P. Fischelis, E. N. Gathercoal, Otto Raubenheimer, and Wilbur L. Scoville.

Reflecting the changing practice of pharmacy, only two other editions of this formulary were issued, the second in 1936 and the third in 1942.

C. TEXTBOOKS AND REFERENCE BOOKS

Pharmacy

C1   MOHR, [Karl Friedrich], 1806–1879 and REDWOOD, Theophilus, 1806–1892

Practical pharmacy: The arrangements, apparatus, and manipulations, of the pharmaceutical shop and laboratory. Edited, with extensive additions, by William Procter, Jr., (1817–1874). Philadelphia: Lea and Blanchard, 1849. xvi, 2, 18–576 p. 14×21 cm. (WU) **AIHP 38**

This first textbook of the art of pharmacy published on American soil was an enlarged adaptation of Redwood's *Practical Pharmacy* (1848). (Redwood had translated and expanded K. F. Mohr's *Lehrbuch der pharmazeutische Technik* (1847) for instructional purposes.) Intended as a handbook for apothecaries and as a text for students, the American edition is illustrated with 500 engravings on wood, and conveys an ideal vision of pharmacy practice in the mid-nineteenth century.

Eighteen chapters describe and explain in detail the apparatus and procedures of practical pharmacy, including such subjects as the arrangement of the pharmaceutical shop and laboratory; weighing and measuring, and specific gravity; sources and management of heat; the processing of crude drugs; preparation of solutions, extracts, tinctures, and fixed oils used in pharmacy; extemporaneous preparations; and reagents.

Only one edition of the book was published.

When William Procter, Jr., edited this book he was professor of pharmacy in the Philadelphia College of Pharmacy, the first pharmacist to occupy that position in an American school of pharmacy (1846). Born in Baltimore, Procter was a pharmacy apprentice in Philadelphia at age fourteen; graduated from the Philadelphia College of Pharmacy in 1837, and three years later was elected a member of the College. In addition to his work as teacher, experimenter, and author, he practiced retail pharmacy for many years. For his many contributions to the profession of pharmacy, including an outstanding role in the founding of the American Pharmaceutical Association, and service as editor of the *American Journal of Pharmacy* (1850–1871), he has been acclaimed as "the father of American pharmacy."

Karl Friedrich Mohr was a German pharmacist and inventor of pharmaceutical and chemical apparatus. (His first name was misrepresented as "Francis" on the titlepage of Procter's American version.) English pharmacist Theophilus Redwood was editor of the *Pharmaceutical Journal* and professor of chemistry and pharmacy at the Pharmaceutical Society of Great Britain.

C2   PARRISH, Edward, 1822–1872

An introduction to practical pharmacy. Designed as a text-book for the student and as a guide to the physician and pharmaceutist with many formulas and prescriptions. Philadelphia: Blanchard & Lea, 1856. v–xxiv, 18–544 p. 14.5×22 cm. (WU) **AIHP 49**

Succeeding Mohr-Redwood-Procter's *Practical Pharmacy* (see C1), Edward Parrish's book, dedicated to Procter, was the first original pharmacy textbook by an American author. Like its predecessor, it was essentially a descriptive text for study and practice, with little theoretical subject matter. Although intended primarily as an introduction to pharmacy for medical students, it did not overlook the students of pharmacy.

It is organized in five parts, with 243 illustrations, and three introductory chapters. Part I deals with the furniture and implements of the dispensing office or shop, weights and measures and specific gravity, and the pharmacopoeia. Part II covers galenical pharmacy in fourteen chapters, including the collection and drying of plants, with emphasis on unofficinal preparations. Part III is devoted, in nine chapters, to the pharmacy of plants and their products, classified in terms of chemical composition. The essentials of inorganic medicinals are treated in nine chapters in Part IV. Part V contains practical directions for prescribing, selecting, combining, and dispensing medications, illustrated by numerous formulas or prescriptions selected from several medical practitioners, and special material on prescription writing.

Current works on materia medica and pharmacy were used as sources, including Garrod's *Essentials of Materia Medica*, Dorvault's *l'Officine*, Pereira's *Materia Medica and Therapeutics*, and Wood and Bache's *United States Dispensatory* (see A4). There were four later editions of *Introduction to Practical Pharmacy* (1859, 1864, 1874, 1884), the title of the third was changed to *A Treatise on Pharmacy*, and the fourth and fifth were edited by Thomas S. Wiegand after Parrish's death.

Born in Philadelphia, Edward Parrish was apprenticed to his brother in 1838 and graduated from the Philadelphia College of Pharmacy in 1842. Upon graduation he started a School of Practical Pharmacy in a drugstore adjoining the University of Pennsylvania to offer instruction in pharmacy to medical students, and later (1850) to pharmacy students also. He taught materia medica (1864–1867) and the theory and practice of pharmacy (from 1867 until his death) at the Philadelphia College of Pharmacy. A founding member of the American Pharmaceutical Association, Parrish held the positions of recording secretary (1853), first vice president (1866), and president (1868).

C3 SWERINGEN, H[iram] V., 1844–1912

Pharmaceutical lexicon: A dictionary of pharmaceutical science. Containing a concise explanation of the various subjects and terms of pharmacy . . . designed as a guide for the pharmaceutist, druggist, physician, etc. Philadelphia: Lindsay & Blakiston, 1873. vi, 576 p. 14×21 cm. (WU) **AIHP 71**

This pharmaceutical dictionary was the first work of its kind in American pharmacy. Planned as a ready reference to facilitate the study of the current *Dispensatory of the United States* and a general understanding of scientific pharmacy, it was intended for pharmacists, "mercantile druggists," physicians, and pharmaceutical students and apprentices.

This compilation draws on the works of many authors including George Wood and Franklin Bache, Edward Parrish, William Procter, Jr., John Maisch, and John Attfield, and offers a wide range of information in abridged form. The first part, nearly 430 pages in dictionary format, explains concisely the subjects and terms of pharmacy. The second part contains, in approximately 140 pages, formulas for officinal, empirical, and dietetic preparations; selections from the prescriptions of the most eminent European and American physicians; an alphabetical list of diseases and their definitions; an account of the modes in use for the preservation of dead bodies for interment or dissection; tables of signs and abbreviations, weights and measures, doses, antidotes to poisons, boiling points of various substances, pharmaceutical equivalents, etc.; and as an item of curiosity, a few leaves of a seventeenth-century dispensatory.

A second edition was published in 1883 under the title *A Dictionary of Pharmaceutical Sciences.*

A native of Navarre, Ohio, Hiram Van Sweringen moved to Fort Wayne, Indiana, in 1858 and lived there until his death. He began working in a drugstore at age sixteen, and it was while connected with the drug business that he entered the practice of medicine before obtaining a medical diploma. He graduated from the Jefferson Medical College in Philadelphia in 1876, returned to Fort Wayne, and was soon in the front rank of medical men in the state of Indiana. Two years later he became professor of materia medica and therapeutics at Fort Wayne Medical College. In recognition of his high standing in the medical profession, he received a master of arts degree from Monmouth College of Illinois.

C4   Boericke, F. E., b. 1829

Three lectures on homoeopathic pharmaceutics. New York and Philadelphia: Boericke and Tafel, [c. 1878]. 1 *l*, 3–49 p. 13×21.5 cm. (WU) **AIHP 05**

Delivered several years earlier to classes at the Homoeopathic Medical College of Pennsylvania, the three lectures in this pamphlet were a distinctive pharmaceutical addition to the American homeopathic literature. Explaining the basics of general homeopathic pharmaceutics, these lectures were meant to enable homeopathic physicians to make their own tinctures, triturations, and dilutions, and to distinguish the fraudulent product from the authentic.

The first lecture explains the principles of preparing medicines and outlines the inert substances used to develop the potency of drugs or to preserve or administer medicines. The second deals with the transformation of drugs into homeopathic remedies by trituration. The third lecture outlines the preparation of solutions and tinctures.

Born in Germany and having completed a literary education in Prussia, Francis E. Boericke emigrated to the United States. He graduated from the Homoeopathic College of Pennsylvania in 1863 at the age of thirty-four, and subsequently lectured on homeopathic pharmaceutics at the Hahnemann College of Philadelphia. He held an M.D. degree, but actively practiced pharmacy, not medicine. His establishment has been described as the best and largest homeopathic pharmacy in the United States. For about fourteen years (1869–1883) he was in partnership in a pharmaceutical and publishing enterprise with Adolf J. Tafel, under the name Boericke and Tafel. In 1883 he established the Hahnemann Publishing House and devoted himself exclusively to the publication of homeopathic works.

C5 REMINGTON, Joseph P[rice], 1847–1918

> The practice of pharmacy: A treatise on the modes of making and dispensing officinal, unofficinal, and extemporaneous preparations, with descriptions of their properties, uses, and doses. Intended as a handbook for pharmacists and physicians and a text-book for students. Philadelphia and London: J. B. Lippincott Co., 1886. 1 *l*, 3–1080 p. 14×20.5 cm. (WU) **AIHP 63**

When this book appeared, the fifth edition of Parrish's *Introduction to Practical Pharmacy* (see C2) and the much older Mohr-Redwood-Procter *Practical Pharmacy* (see C1) were the dominant American pharmacy textbooks. But Joseph Remington's work included current improvements in apparatus, new processes and preparations, new discoveries in theoretical and applied chemistry and physics, and a different arrangement and treatment of the subject matter. By organizing the text from the elementary to the advanced, with the subjects following one another in a natural order, Remington introduced the prototype of the modern American pharmacy textbook.

Intended as a text for students and as a handbook for pharmacists and physicians, the book is divided into six parts, with nearly 500 illustrations. Part I (twenty chapters) includes detailed descriptions of apparatus, and definitions and comments on general pharmaceutical procedures. Part II (eleven chapters) covers the preparations of U.S.P. VI. Part III (seventeen chapters) deals with inorganic chemical substances, giving precedence to officinal preparations. It includes also a systematic tabulation of descriptions, solubilities, and tests for identity and impurities; chemical operations are accompanied by equations and reactions are explained in words. Part IV (fourteen chapters) covers organic chemical substances, grouped according to the physical and medical properties of their principal constituents. Part V (five chapters) is devoted to extemporaneous pharmacy. Part VI contains a formulary of unofficinal preparations most likely to be requested, which were of rather difficult accessibility, or that had been deleted from old revisions of the *United States Pharmacopoeia*.

Other more concise American textbooks followed this treatise in the last decade of the nineteenth century. The most widely known were *The Beginnings of Pharmacy* (Reinhold Rother, 1887, 342 p.), an entirely different type of elementary handbook; *Handbook of Pharmacy* (Virgil Coblentz, 1894, 480 p.), a text for systematic study and a reference guide for daily consultation; and *A Treatise on Pharmacy for Students and Pharmacists* (Charles Caspari, Jr., 1895, 679 p.), of the same scope and purpose as Coblentz's book, but with more emphasis on pharmaceutical chemistry. But only Remington's work has persisted through several revisions (e.g., see C9), and under the title *Remington's Pharmaceutical Sciences* is at present a popular encyclopedic treatise.

Born in Philadelphia, Joseph Price Remington graduated from the Philadelphia College of Pharmacy in 1866. After serving in manufacturing and community pharmacy, he became associated with the Philadelphia College of Pharmacy. This association continued for nearly fifty years, with Remington beginning as assistant to Edward Parrish (1871) and William Procter, Jr. (1872), then as professor of theory and practice of pharmacy (1874), and as dean from 1893 until his death. A member of the Committee of Revision of the *United States Pharmacopoeia* for over four decades, he was the first vice-chairman when the noted Sixth Revision (see B7) and the Seventh Revision were issued, was elected chairman for the Eighth Revision (see B14), and continued in the chairmanship until his death.

Remington joined the American Pharmaceutical Association soon after graduation and promptly became prominent in its activities. With a worldwide reputation, he held membership in many honorary and professional societies in the United States and abroad. His memory is perpetuated in the Remington Honor Medal, instituted by the New York branch of the American Pharmaceutical Association in 1919, as the first national honorary award for distinguished services in American pharmacy.

C6 SCOVILLE, Wilbur L[incoln], 1865–1942

The art of compounding. A textbook for students and a reference book for pharmacists and the prescription counter. Philadelphia: P. Blakiston Son & Co., 1895. 1 *l*, 5–264 p. 15×22.5 cm. (ICRL) **AIHP 69**

This book is one of the earliest and best known examples of textbooks specializing in the theory and practice of filling prescriptions. Issued at a time when the literature on this subject was widely scattered, it was meant as a textbook for students and a reference book for pharmacists.

Of fourteen chapters varying in length, the more extensive, which comprise about three-quarters of the text, are: "The Prescription,"

"Mixtures," "Emulsions," "Pills," "Powders," "Ointments, Cerates, and Plasters," and "Incompatibility." Other chapters deal with nomenclature and homeopathic pharmacy, and with such pharmaceutical preparations as confections, electuaries, and jellies; lozenges, troches, bacills, tablets, pastils and lamels; suppositories; poultices, plasmas, pencils, and medicated dressings.

In presenting the subject matter, the general text explaining the underlying principles is followed by prescriptions illustrating their application, as well as methods of mixing, the physical properties of the substances used, and in some degree, the range and variety of extemporaneous pharmacy.

The book went through nine editions, the last one in 1957. A more concise contemporary text was *Prescription Practice and General Dispensing: An Elementary Treatise for Students of Pharmacy* (J. H. Beal, 1908). These elementary texts were replaced with the first edition of Husa's *Pharmaceutical Dispensing*, 1935 (see C11).

Born in Connecticut, Wilbur Lincoln Scoville graduated from the Massachusetts College of Pharmacy and was professor of pharmacy at that institution from 1892 to 1904. He was associated with Parke, Davis & Company for nearly three decades, as research pharmacist from 1907, and as head of the analytical department from 1924 until his retirement in 1934. A member of the Committee of Revision of the *United States Pharmacopoeia* (1900–1910, 1920–1940), he was also a member of the Committee of Revision that issued the second through fifth editions of the *National Formulary*, and served as its chairman for the fourth edition. Scoville received honorary degrees from the Massachusetts College of Pharmacy, the University of Michigan, and Columbia University, and was awarded the Ebert Prize in 1923 and the Remington Medal in 1929.

C7 WALL, Otto A., 1846–1922

The prescription, therapeutically, pharmaceutically, grammatically and historically considered. Third edition. St. Louis: Aug. Gast Bank Note and Litho. Co., 1898. 2 *l*, 211 p. 13.5×19 cm. (WU) **AIHP 76**

The first edition of this book was published under the title *The Prescription Therapeutically, Pharmaceutically and Gramatically Considered* (St. Louis, MO, 1888). Adapted to U.S.P. VI (1880), and written from a physician's viewpoint, it was an early attempt to offer theoretical and practical knowledge on prescription-writing to American pharmacists as well as to physicians. The third edition is presented here because, with the introduction of corrections and additions, it represents a significant improvement over the first and second editions. Moreover, it deals with general principles not adapted to any particular pharmacopoeia.

The book is divided into five parts. Part I deals with general considerations such as the meaning and classification of prescriptions, the definitions and descriptions of thirty-nine dosage forms, observations on patent and proprietary medicines, and the manner of writing permanent prescriptions (i.e., formulas). Part II covers weights and measures, including systems of numeration, the necessity of an international system of weights, and the metric system. Part III is essentially an elementary course in prescription Latin, of which the author was a strong advocate. Part IV deals extensively with extemporaneous prescriptions, covering such topics as components of the prescription, combination of remedies, doses, the act of prescribing, influences modifying the action of medicines, and incompatibilities. Eleven solid and nine liquid dosage forms are described in this part and illustrated with specific formulations. Part V is a superficial, though interesting, history of the prescription. This is followed by a six-page appendix on the origin of the ℞ symbol, which adds to information previously given in the text. Four editions were published (to 1917) and it was one of the sources for Bernard Fantus's *Text Book on Prescription-Writing* (see C10).

When Otto Augustus Wall published this book, he was professor of materia medica, pharmacognosy, and botany at the St. Louis College of Pharmacy, a position he held for over forty years beginning in 1873. Born in St. Louis, Missouri, he received his education at the St. Louis College of Pharmacy (Ph.G., 1868) and at the Missouri Medical College (M.D., 1870).

Most widely known as a teacher, Wall also practiced medicine for several years (until 1882), and manufactured pharmaceuticals for a short period. Other professional activities included membership in the American Pharmaceutical Association and on the Committee of Revision of the U.S.P. (1880–1900); and serving as vice president of the U.S.P. Convention (1900–1910).

His other publications include *A Companion to the United States Pharmacopoeia* (with Oscar Oldberg, 1884), *Elementary Lessons in Latin* (1900 and 1917), and *Handbook of Pharmacognosy* (five editions from 1897 to 1928).

C8 RUDDIMAN, Edsel A., 1864–1954

Incompatibilities in prescriptions for students in pharmacy and medicine and practicing pharmacists and physicians. New York: John Wiley & Sons; London: Chapman & Hall, 1899. 1 *l*, 1 p., iii, 264 p. 13.5×20.5 cm. (WU) **AIHP 66**

As the first compendium published in the United States devoted exclusively to the identification and explanation of the more common pharmaceutical incompatibilities, this book draws upon at least twenty-six sources, including pharmaceutical journals, texts like Caspari's *Treatise on Pharmacy* and Scoville's *Art of Compounding* (see C6), the United States and National dispensatories (see A4), the *United States Pharmacopoeia*, books on chemical analysis and on materia medica, and the *Proceedings* of the American Pharmaceutical Association (see C46).

The text is arranged in two parts. The first section discusses at length the more probable chemical and pharmaceutical incompatibilities of the most important natural and chemical drugs, arranged alphabetically by their Latin names. The second part contains over 300 sample prescriptions which test a student's ability to find and remedy existing incompatibilities, before referring to explanatory notes given at the end of the book.

The most popular work of its kind, *Incompatibilities in Prescriptions* was issued in 1897 and reprinted in 1899. Six editions were published, the last one in 1936.

Edsel Alexander Ruddiman was born in Michigan and earned degrees from the University of Michigan (Ph.C., 1886 and Ph.M., 1887) and from Vanderbilt University (M.D., 1893). For about thirty years (1890–1920) he taught materia medica and pharmacy at Vanderbilt University, serving as dean of the school of pharmacy for one year. He also served as chemist to the Tennessee Board of Pharmacy (1897–1920) and as food and drug inspector (1907–1914). Later, for sixteen years, he was a research chemist with the Ford Motor Company. His other publications include *Why's in Pharmacy* (1906), *Manual of Materia Medica* (1907), and *Theoretical and Practical Pharmacy* (1917).

C9	REMINGTON, Joseph P[rice], 1847–1918

The practice of pharmacy: A treatise on the modes of making and dispensing official, unofficial, and extemporaneous preparations, with descriptions of medicinal substances, their properties, uses and doses. Intended as a hand-book for pharmacists and physicians and a text-book for students. Fifth edition. Philadelphia and London: J. B. Lippincott Co., 1907. 2 *l*, iii–xxv, 1541 p. 15×24 cm. (WU) **AIHP 64**

The fifth edition of Remington's *The Practice of Pharmacy* is representative of a work with lasting influence. Other pharmacy textbooks published in the United States in the early 1900s reflected in some degree the predominance of earlier editions of this work (see C5). This edition reflects the changes of U.S.P. VIII (see B14) and of N.F. III after they became legal standards. A unique feature, introduced in the third edition, omitted in the fourth, and re-introduced in the fifth, is a list of questions for the use of home students in revising their work and for state boards of pharmacy in framing examination questions.

In the same pattern of the first edition, but one and a half times larger, the fifth edition is arranged in six parts and has over 800 illustrations. Part I (twenty chapters) consists of extensive descriptions of pharmaceutical procedures and apparatus. Part II (eleven chapters) covers U.S.P. VIII and some unofficial preparations under chapter headings such as aqueous solutions, alcoholic solutions, ethereal solutions, and aqueous liquids made by percolation and maceration. Part III (seventeen chapters) deals with official and unofficial inorganic preparations. Part IV (fourteen chapters) treats the official and some unofficial organic medicinals, classified according to their chemical nature, and includes a chapter on pharmaceutical testing. Part V (six chapters), titled "Magistral Pharmacy," discusses the topics of dispensing, prescriptions, liquid and solid extemporaneous preparations, incompatibility, and solid extemporaneous preparations used externally. Part VI includes a summary of changes in N.F. III, answers to practical problems and exercises, a glossary of uncommon names, terms, and substances, a list of questions, and an index.

Less comprehensive but similar in scope and intent was Henry V. Arny's *Principles of Pharmacy* (Philadelphia, 1909), a textbook aimed at explaining the pharmacopoeia from its pharmaceutical viewpoint, which went through four editions (to 1937).

For a biographical sketch of this master pharmacist of the late nineteenth and early twentieth centuries, see C5.

C10 FANTUS, Bernard, 1874–1940

A text book on prescription-writing and pharmacy with practice in prescription-writing, laboratory exercises in pharmacy and a reference list of the official drugs especially designed for medical students. Second edition. Chicago: Chicago Medical Book Co., 1913. iii-xii, 404 p. 14.5×22.5 cm. (WU) **AIHP 17**

The first edition of this volume appeared under the title *Laboratory Manual on Pharmacognosy, Pharmacy and Prescription Writing* (Chicago, 1902), and was intended as a laboratory handbook for medical students taking their first materia medica course. The second and final edition is presented here because it gives more emphasis to the principles and "the art of prescription-writing." Its purpose was to teach medical students a first level course on the best form in which medicines could be prescribed. Fantus believed that without proper training in this area, "the young practitioner falls readily into the trap set for him by the proprietary medicine merchant." A combination textbook and laboratory manual, this book illustrates the prescribing practices expected of physicians, and hence the dispensing practices that pharmacists would be called upon to perform. Published in 1913 but copyrighted and prefaced in 1905, this edition is more detailed and authoritative than Wall's *The Prescription*, a book published a few years earlier (see C7), that served as one of its sources. Some twenty works were consulted freely, including U.S.P. VIII, the *United States Dispensatory*, Remington's *Practice of Pharmacy*, Scoville's *Art of Compounding*, and Ruddiman's *Incompatibilities in Prescriptions*.

A *Text Book on Prescription-Writing* has three parts, each one divided into chapters with many subheadings. Part I, Prescription-Writing, in five chapters, covers definitions, form and language of prescriptions, the determination of quantities, the composition of prescriptions, and prescription ethics. Such topics as parts of the prescription, rules for time and frequent administration, methods of writing a prescription, and the prescribing of placebos are discussed. Part II, Pharmacy, discusses forty individual dosage forms grouped under four orders according to properties: non-extractive liquid preparations, extractive preparations, solid preparations for internal use, and external preparations. The orders are divided into suborders, divisions and classes (dosage forms). Each class or dosage form is described under its Latin and English names, including such information as abbreviations, gender, pronunciation, definition, doses, uses, and official (U.S.P. VIII) preparations. Problem-solving, exercises in prescription-writing and laboratory exercises complement most of the monographs. Part III is a reference list, for prescribing U.S.P. VIII drugs and preparations. The book has a table of contents, an appendix giving suggestions for the laboratory exercises, and an index.

Physician Bernard Fantus was professor of pharmacology and therapeutics at the University of Illinois College of Medicine when he published *A Text Book on Prescription-Writing*. A native of Hungary, Fantus received part of his education in Vienna, Strassburg and Berlin, and M.D. and M.S. degrees in Illinois (1899) and Michigan (1917), respectively. His long academic career included teaching courses in materia medica and therapeutics, and in clinical medicine at the Rush Medical College of Chicago, and lecturing at the University of Illinois School of Pharmacy.

His professional activities included membership in the American Pharmaceutical Association, the American Medical Association, the Society of Internal Medicine, and in the revision committees of the U.S.P. and N.F., and serving as editor of *General Therapeutics*. In addition to his interest in the improvement of prescription writing, he made contributions to the technique of medication, focusing on pharmaceuticals such as Fuller's Earth, candy medications, antidotes for mercuric chloride, and useful cathartics. As Medical Director of the Cook County Hospital in Chicago, he was a leader in the establishment of blood banks in hospitals.

His other publications include *Essentials of Prescription Writing* (1906) and *The Technic of Medication* (1926). The latter consists of reprints from the *Journal of the American Medical Association*, and went through three editions to 1938.

C11 HUSA, William J., 1896–1985

Pharmaceutical dispensing. A textbook for students of pharmaceutical compounding and dispensing. Easton, PA: Mack Printing Co., Printers, 1935. 1 *l*, v–vii, 1 *l*, 428 p. 15×21 cm. (WU) **AIHP 26**

Replacing an earlier elementary approach to pharmaceutical dispensing (see C6), this book introduced a scientific and professional treatment of the art of compounding and dispensing, including a comprehensive study of incompatibilities. An invaluable source of information about prescriptions of the 1930s, *Pharmaceutical Dispensing* contains over 1250 prescriptions of various types obtained from "professional," neighborhood, chain, and hospital pharmacies located in small towns, medium sized cities, and large urban centers of the United States. The author intended this work primarily as a textbook for students, and as aid for teachers and pharmacists. He compiled this volume drawing from his experience of over twenty years as a retail pharmacist, teacher and researcher. In selecting the material, he covered all of the topics related to pharmaceutical dispensing in *The Pharmaceutical Syllabus* (fourth edition, 1932) and in *Basic Material for a Pharmaceutical Curriculum* (1927). (See C48 and C50.)

The first of thirty-five chapters deals with the general features of prescriptions. Chapters II–XV discuss different types of prescriptions such as powders, capsules and cachets, tablet triturates and compressed tablets, lozenges and pastilles, pills, suppositories, ointments, dermatologic pastes and other external preparations, emulsions, and solutions. Reflecting the transformation taking place in the materia medica, many proprietary specialties appear in these prescriptions. Of three chapters dealing with incompatibilities, chapter XVI presents the classifications of incompatibilities and general methods to avoid or overcome them. Chapters XVII and XVIII discuss inorganic and organic incompatibilities, respectively, classifying the drugs according to their physical and chemical properties, thus bringing together those having similar incompatibilities.

Evincing the already changing profile of the dispensing function, *Pharmaceutical Dispensing* includes subjects not traditionally covered in texts of this kind. For example, the last fourteen chapters contain such topics as receiving the prescription, finishing the prescription, checking the finished prescription, legal aspects of prescriptions, prescription pricing, delivery of the prescription, professional pharmacy, the reference library of the retail pharmacy, detailing the doctor, the place of clinical laboratory work in professional pharmacy, and hospital pharmacy.

Used as a textbook during at least forty years, the modification in scope, purpose, and title of later editions of the book reflect the evolution occurring in the practice of pharmacy. For instance, the subtitle of the fifth edition (*Husa's Pharmaceutical Dispensing*, 1959), edited by Eric W. Martin, in part read " . . . a reference book for pharmacists in retail and hospital pharmacy and in pharmaceutical development and production." The subtitle of the seventh edition, *Dispensing of Medication* (1971), also edited by Martin, is indicative of this change: "A manual on the formulation of pharmaceutical products, the dispensing of prescriptions and the professional practice of pharmacy."

A native of Iowa City, Iowa, William J. Husa received degrees from the University of Iowa (Ph.G., B.A., and Ph.D.) and from Columbia University (M.A.). He was the first professor of pharmacy and head of the Department of Pharmacy of the University of Florida School of Pharmacy, holding these positions from c. 1923 until his retirement in 1961. When he wrote this book, he drew on experiences of more than twenty years as a retail pharmacist, teacher, and researcher in industrial and academic laboratories. He was vice-chairman of the National Conference of Pharmaceutical Research (see C51), chairman of this organization's Committee on Pharmaceutical Dispensing, and past chairman of the Scientific Section of the American Pharmaceutical Association. Later on he served as chairman of the Section on Practical Pharmacy and Dispensing of the Association and as chairman of the Conference (1938–1944).

Materia Medica, Pharmacognosy, Pharmacology and Therapeutics

Materia Medica

C12 CULLEN, William, 1710–1790

Lectures on the materia medica as delivered by William Cullen, M.D., professor of medicine in the University of Edinburgh. Now published by permission of the author, and with many corrections from the collation of different manuscripts by the editors. Philadelphia: Robert Bell, Printer, 1775. viii, 512 p. 19×24 cm. (Evans 14000) (WU) **AIHP 08**

The earliest treatise on materia medica printed in America, *Lectures on the Materia Medica*, was authored by one of the best-known therapists of the eighteenth century. It was a reprint of a 1773 London edition, with the difference that corrections that had been listed at the end of the London edition were inserted in their proper places in the American edition. The London edition was based on a course of lectures delivered in Edinburgh in 1761, and became the predecessor of the author's better-known *A Treatise of the Materia Medica* (Edinburgh, 1781 and Philadelphia, 1789).

The *Lectures* influenced other works appearing later in the United States (e.g., C13). Illustrative of eighteenth-century therapeutics, the book uses Latin and English titles to describe over 600 vegetable, animal, and mineral substances classified into twenty therapeutic categories, including nutrients, astringents, emollients, stimulants, sedatives, expectorants, and others. Reflecting Cullen's advocacy for dietary prescriptions, most substances, either "natural or prepared by art," are explained in a detailed narrative style under four topics: their cognition and distinction from other articles of the materia medica, their dietary or medicinal virtues, the basis of their dietary or medicinal virtues, so far as could be perceived in their visible or chemical qualities, and their pharmaceutical treatment and other circumstances necessary for their application in medicine or diet, explaining that the action of medicines depends on their own nature and on the specific condition of the system to which they are applied. The pharmaceutical treatment is limited to an indication of the forms in which some of the drugs had to be used, such as decoctions, infusions, and spirits. The book includes Cullen's "Catalog of the Materia Medica" and an index. A second edition was published in 1808.

Born in Scotland, William Cullen apprenticed as an apothecary and received an M.D. degree at Glasgow in 1740, where he subsequently practiced and lectured on medicine. From 1775 until his death he was on the Edinburgh medical faculty, becoming one of the greatest clinicians of the eighteenth century. Although his pathology was founded on a neurosis theory of disease, his therapeutics were more traditional. An eclectic, more specifically a Hippocratist, he prescribed diets, favoring vegetables, milk and fish. As for drugs, he advocated the use of opium, wine, and camphor, as well as metallic medicaments.

C13 MURRAY, J[ohn], 1778–1820

Elements of materia medica and pharmacy. Two vols.
in one. Philadelphia: B. and T. Kite, 1808. vi–xii, 13–447
p. 12.5×20 cm. (Evans 15670) (WU) **AIHP 39**

Originally published in Edinburgh in 1804, this is probably the
first American edition of a book on materia medica to include general
principles of "pharmaceutic chemistry," i.e., pharmaceutical operations and general chemical analysis of the materia medica. A lecturer
on materia medica and pharmacy, Murray wrote this book to render
his lectures more useful, since "there is no elementary work on Pharmacy, in which the discoveries of modern chemistry are introduced:
and former systems of materia medica . . . have in some measure
become obsolete and deficient, in consequence of the changes that
have taken place . . . in the theory and practice of medicine, and in
the sciences with which it is connected."

Modifying Cullen's twenty-class arrangement of the materia
medica (see C12), Murray introduces a twenty-one-class system that
includes new classes, such as narcotics and anthelmintics, deletes
others like nutrients and stimulants, and has thirteen classes in common with Cullen's classification. In addition, some of the principles
of pharmaceutical processing are revised. Thacher adopted these innovations in his *American New Dispensatory* (see A3).

The first volume consists of an introduction and two parts. The
introduction covers the objectives of the materia medica and pharmacy; Part I deals with pharmaceutical operations and general chemical analysis of the materia medica; and Part II includes over 200
medicinal substances classified into twenty-one therapeutic classes,
such as narcotics, tonics, emetics, diuretics, and diluents. Each medicinal substance is described under its Latin name in terms of its
natural history, physical properties, chemical analysis, pharmaceutical processing, uses, doses, and modes of administration; its officinal
preparations are given also. The second volume (Part III, about half
the book) is devoted to the pharmaceutical preparations of the *Edinburgh Pharmacopoeia* (ninth edition, 1803), with corresponding preparations of the *London Pharmacopoeia* (1788) and some non-phar-
macopoeial preparations used in practice. It has twenty-five chapters
under headings such as preparations of simple medicines, conserves,
tinctures, oily preparations, powders, and ointments. It also has two
appendices covering gases, electricity and galvanism, and prescriptions and doses. The book ends with a table of changed names in
the Edinburgh and London pharmacopoeias, and English and Latin
indices.

An enlarged edition, similar in content and organization, appeared under the title *A System of Materia Medica and Pharmacy*

(1815), with notes by Nathaniel Chapman, a professor of materia medica at the University of Pennsylvania. It was followed in 1828 by a further enlarged and rearranged edition under the same title, with notes and additions by John B. Beck, professor of materia medica at the University of New York.

Physician John Murray was lecturer on chemistry, and on materia medica and pharmacy in Edinburgh and a Fellow of the Royal College of Physicians, of the Royal Society of Edinburgh, and of the Geological Society of London.

C14 BARTON, Benjamin Smith, 1766–1815

Collections for an essay towards a materia medica of the United States. Third edition. Philadelphia: Edward Earle and Co., 1810. Part first: 2 l, v–vi, 3–67 p. Part second: 1 l, iii–xv, 53 p. 12.5×21 cm. (Evans 19478) (WU) **AIHP 02**

The first comprehensive work on American indigenous medicinal plants by an American author, this book was originally published in two parts—"Part First" in 1798, with a second edition in 1801 (December), and "Part Second" in 1804. It is presented here in the somewhat improved and enlarged third edition (December 1810) in which, for the first time, both parts of the book—the 1801 and the 1804 editions—are brought together.

Intended as a guide for the study of the nature and medicinal properties of the native flora, the book includes fifty-nine plants, all native (except one) and all medicinal (except two). It is arranged in nine sections: I Astringents, II Tonics, III Stimulants, IV Errhines, V Sialagoga, VI Emetics, VII Cathartics, VIII Diuretics, IX Anthelmintics. Written in a narrative style, "The facts and observations . . . are thrown together with too little regard to method, to give it a claim to the title of an ESSAY." Under the Latin name of each plant is given information such as: description, common and botanical name, habitat, medicinal properties, therapeutic uses and how used (e.g., decoction of the roots), and plants of comparable properties and uses. Their pharmaceutical treatment is not considered.

This book was the main source on indigenous plants for Thacher's *American New Dispensatory* (see A3).

Benjamin Smith Barton was one of America's foremost botanists, a so-called "father of American materia medica." A native of Pennsylvania, he studied in Edinburgh and London, and at the age of twenty-three years received an M.D. degree from Göttingen. In 1789, the year of his graduation, he was appointed professor of natural history and botany in the College of Philadelphia. Later, he was professor of materia medica, natural history, and botany in the University of Pennsylvania, where his encouragement of research on the medicinal properties of American plants was evident in many graduate theses. He was a member of a committee on pharmacopoeia appointed by the College of Physicians of Philadelphia to compile material on pharmaceutical substances and processes. Author of several books on botany, and many articles on medicine, history and archaeology, his revision of William Cullen's *Treatise of the Materia Medica* (see C12) appeared under the title *Professor Cullen's Treatise of the Materia Medica*, in 1812.

C15 BARTON, William P[aul] C[rillon], 1786–1856

Vegetable materia medica of the United States, or medical botany: containing a botanical, general, and medical history of medicinal plants indigenous to the United States. Illustrated by coloured engravings made after original drawings from nature, done by the author. Two vols. Philadelphia: M. Carey & Son, vol. 1 1817; vol. 2 1818. Vol. 1: 3 *l*, vi–xv, 17–273 p. 21×26.5 cm. Vol 2: 3 *l*, viii–xvi, 9–243 p. 21×26.5 cm. (Evans 40143) (WU) **AIHP 03**

Cultivating his famous uncle's concern for the study of medical botany (Benjamin S. Barton, see C14), William P. C. Barton initiated with this book the description and drawing of indigenous medicinal plants in the United States, as an incentive for the study and observation of native plants by physicians and botanists.

In no particular sequence, the book describes fifty plants—twenty-four in the first volume and twenty-six in the second—including full-page color engravings made from original drawings by the author, and sketches of the flowers and fruits. Each description includes the botanical name, popular English synonyms, references to scientific works cited, best specific character, a brief account of its pharmaceutical preparations, medical properties, uses and doses, chemical analysis (if any had been made), economical uses, and an explanation of the plates and sketches.

Praised as "an excellent account of our medicinal plants," this work influenced other books appearing shortly after, such as Jacob Dyckman's *Edinburgh New Dispensatory* (New York, 1818) and William Zollickoffer's *A Materia Medica of the United States* (Baltimore, 1819). Closely related in character and scope was *American Medical Botany* (Boston, three volumes, 1817–1820), by the renowned physician and botanist Jacob Bigelow.

The author, William Paul Crillon Barton, member of a distinguished scientific and professional family, studied medicine at the University of Pennsylvania under his uncle Benjamin Smith Barton. W. P. C. Barton taught botany at that institution, and materia medica at the Jefferson Medical School. He was a systematic and accurate botanist, and among his other publications is the beautifully illustrated *Flora of North America*, 1821–23.

C16 PARIS, John Ayrton, 1785–1856

Pharmacologia; or the history of medicinal substances, with a view to establish the art of prescribing and of composing extemporaneous formulae upon fixed and scientific principles; illustrated by formulae, in which the intention of each element is designated by key letters. From the last London edition, with a general English index. New York: F. & R. Lockwood, 1822. 1 *l*, iii–xii, 1 *l*, 15–428 p. 14×22 cm. (WU) **AIHP 48**

Intended for practitioners and students, this book was the first attempt in the United States, as it had been earlier in England, to discuss the basic principles of compounding prescriptions, to illustrate the principles with formulas, and to explain the role of the ingredients in the general scheme of the formulas. The first American edition, in two parts, was based on the fourth London edition (1820) of the same title. A general English index was added to the American edition.

Distinguishing the terms *pharmacologia* (scientific methods of administering medicines) and *pharmacopoeia* (processes for preparing medicines), the book deals only with the former. The first part covers the subject of medicinal combination, illustrating its principles in formulas written in Latin. The second part consists of the medicinal history and chemical properties of the entities that form the combinations. This part is arranged in alphabetical sequence, "not only as being best calculated for reference, but one which, in an elementary work at least, is less likely to mislead, than any arrangement founded in their medicinal powers." Under each item appears information such as physical characteristics, chemical composition or the constituents responsible for its medicinal activity, relative solubility, incompatible substances, specific doses, medicinal uses and effects, officinal and extemporaneous preparations, and adulterations. For preparations, the *London Pharmacopoeia* was the preferred source, with occasional reference to the pharmacopoeias of Edinburgh and Dublin.

An interesting feature of this book is the inclusion of formulas for "quack medicines" at the end of the entry for the particular substance that constitutes its main ingredient, because "it is essential that the practitioner should be acquainted with their composition, for . . . it is but too probable that he may be called upon to counteract its [i.e., a quack medicine's] baneful influence." About 144 patent medicines and nostrums are included, such as Barclay's Antibilious Pills, Cheltenham Salts, and Davidson's Remedy for Cancer.

A second American edition, based on the fifth London edition (1822), was published in two volumes (1823–24), with additions and illustrations of the materia medica of the United States by Ansel W. Ives, Fellow of the College of Physicians and Surgeons of the University of the State of New York. This edition has an expanded list of 166 patent medicines. The ninth London edition (1843), published in New York in 1844 with notes by physician C. A. Lee, has been described as one of the best textbooks on materia medica.

Physician John Ayrton Paris, a native of Cambridge, England, was president of the Royal College of Physicians from 1844 to his death, Fellow of the Philosophical Society of Cambridge and of the Medical Society of Edinburgh, and senior physician to the Westminster Hospital.

C17 RAFINESQUE, Constantine S[amuel], 1783–1840

Medical flora; or manual of the medical botany of the United States of North America. Two vols. in one. Philadelphia: Atkinson & Alexander, vol. 1 1828; vol. 2 1830. Vol. 1: 1 *l*, xii, 268 p. Vol. 2: 276 p. 10.5×18 cm. (DNLM) **AIHP 62**

This was one of the most popular books of the nineteenth-century medico-botanical movement in the United States. Intended as an "accurate, complete, portable and cheap" reference for "medical students, Physicians, Druggists, Pharmaciens, Chemists, Botanists, Florists, Herbalists, Collectors of herbs, heads of families, Infirmaries, etc.," it was extensively used by all botanic sects, and was a *vade mecum* for their more educated practitioners. Of pharmaceutical and phytochemical importance, it advocated the procurement of effective medicines from plants, under the premise that "the active principles of medical plants may be obtained . . . by chemical operations."

About fifteen years of botanical and medical observations and travels served as background for the book, and the works of many American physicians and botanists were consulted, among them those of Benjamin S. Barton (see C14), W. P. C. Barton and Jacob Bigelow (see C15), James Thacher (see A3), and Peter Smith (see C28).

Medical Flora contains a selection of figures and descriptions of over 100 "of the most active and efficient" medicinal plants, including all the species mentioned in the books of Bigelow and W. P. C. Barton, and notes on nearly 500 equivalent substitutes. Arranged in a numbered alphabetical sequence by botanical names, plants A to H—with fifty-two plates—appear in the first volume; and plants I to Z—with forty-eight plates—appear in the second. Each monograph includes the names (botanical, English, French, German, officinal, common, and synonyms), botanical and medical authorities, generic and specific characters, botanical description, locality or native places of growth, history of the genus and species, physical and chemical properties, medical properties, uses, doses, preparations, and equivalent substitutes.

Only one edition was published.

Born in Turkey of French descent, Constantine Samuel Rafinesque received his education in Europe under private tutors. He conducted botanical explorations in New Jersey and Virginia (1802–04), then moved to Palermo, Sicily, where he exported medicinal plants for ten years (1805–15). After serving as professor of botany, natural history, and modern languages at Transylvania University in Lexington, Kentucky, for seven years (1819–1826), he resided in Philadelphia until his death. Rafinesque lectured at the Franklin Institute for one year (1826–27). A prominent botanist, extensive traveler, and prolific writer, he published books on history, medical botany, and ichthyology.

C18 DUNGLISON, Robley, 1798–1869

New remedies: the method of preparing and administering them; their effects on the health and diseased economy, &c. Philadelphia: Adam Waldie, 1839. 3 *l*, i–viii, 429 p. 14×23 cm. (DNLM) **AIHP 13**

This book is an early example of a literature designed "to enable the [medical] profession to form an accurate estimate of the value of remedies of more recent introduction or of the older remedies whose use has been revived under novel applications."

Citing the British, Italian, German, and French literature, the author gives most credit as a useful source to Victor Adolph Riecke's *Die neuern Arzneimittel . . .* (Stuttgart, 1837). In addition, he apparently was strongly influenced by François Magendie's *Formulaire pour la préparation et l'emploi de plusiers nouveaux médicaments*, which appeared eventually in nine editions and several languages. Dunglison had edited the "First American Edition" of Magendie's work under the title, *Formulary for the Preparation and Mode of Employing Several New Remedies* (Philadelphia, 1824).

New Remedies stresses the alkaloids and glycosides, like Magendie's *Formulaire*, but with a more comprehensive approach. The monographs, usually of three to twelve pages each, offer substantial pharmaceutical information. Arranged alphabetically, each monograph gives official Latin names, synonyms, and the English, French, and German titles, chemical and physical properties, methods and formulas for preparation, medicinal effects, forms of administration, and average doses, and sometimes a bit of history. Following the monographs, a short "Supplement" is devoted to such therapeutic measures as compression, counter-irritation, Galvanism, and injections into the Eustachian tube. Enhancing the usefulness of the book are two indexes, one for remedies and one for diseases.

A native of Keswick, England, Robley Dunglison received a surgical degree at the Royal College of Surgeons (London, 1819) and a medical degree at Erlangen (Bavaria, 1823). In 1824, at the age of twenty-six, and already the author of a treatise on children's diseases and editor of the *London Medical Repository and Medical Intelligencer*, he left England to become the first full-time professor of medicine at the newly established University of Virginia, a position he held for nine years. For over thirty years (until 1868) Dunglison was Professor of the Institutes of Medicine at the Jefferson Medical College in Philadelphia. Having acquired world-wide reputation through his *Human Physiology* (1832) and *Medical Dictionary* (1833), by the time he wrote *New Remedies* he was, in addition to his academic position, attending physician at the Philadelphia Hospital, honorary member of the Philadelphia College of Pharmacy, and fellow of the College of Physicians of Philadelphia. Numerous other publications include a treatise on materia medica (1843) and a book on the practice of medicine (1842).

C19 PAINE, Martyn, 1794–1877

A therapeutical arrangement of the materia medica, or the materia medica arranged upon physiological principles, and in the order of the general practical value which remedial agents hold and their several denominations, and in conformity with the physiological doctrines set forth in the medical and physiological commentaries. New York: J. & H. G. Langley, 1842. 2 *l*, vi–xii, 14–271 p. 11×18.5 cm. (WU) **AIHP 47**

Based on humoral therapy, this book introduced a novel therapeutical and physiological arrangement of the materia medica in which the medicinal substances were classified in classes, orders, and subdivisions. A rather elaborate system, it attempted to give the student a comprehensive view of the merits and physiological relationships of different medicines by establishing their relative therapeutic value within each general denomination, to offer a convenient method of adjusting the doses of medicines, and to indicate which medicines could be most advantageously combined.

The remedial agents (over 900 entries including cross references) are grouped under eleven classes, such as antiflogistics, permanent tonics, diffusible stimulants, anthelmintics, chemical agents, diet and regimen in a general sense, and genito-urinary agents. Within each class there are nine orders. For example, under antiflogistics are bloodletting, cathartics, emetics, and alteratives. Under each order there are various subdivisions, e.g., mercurials, jalap, and castor oil come under cathartics. For each medicinal substance the synonyms, composition, dose, combinations, use, and formula are given under the Latin or English names. The formulas do not indicate the proportions because, "systematic formulae, with definite proportions of the several ingredients purporting to be adapted to diseases of some given *name*, and especially where the compounds may be extemporaneously prepared, are not founded upon just conceptions of pathology, lead others to inaccurate views, and encourage indolence and empiricism." Characters and symbols express the combination of remedies in the formulas. The book has a table of contents and an index.

Born in Vermont, physician Martyn Paine graduated from Harvard University (A.B., 1813 and M.D., 1816). A co-founder of the New York University Medical School, he was professor of the institutes of medicine and materia medica (1840–1850) and of therapeutics and materia medica (1850–1867), then professor emeritus. A prolific contributor to the medical literature, Paine's publications include *Essays on the Philosophy of Vitality* (see C30) and *Materia Medica and Therapeutics* (1848).

C20 GRIFFITH, R. Eglesfeld, 1798–1850

Medical botany: or descriptions of the more important plants used in medicine, with their history, properties, and mode of administration. Philadelphia: Lea and Blanchard, 1847. 2 *l*, vii–xv, [17]–704 p., 16 *l*. 15×23 cm. (WU) **AIHP 20**

This is one of the earliest American treatises to bring together a considerable amount of data on the medicinal history and chemical composition of the foreign and domestic vegetable materia medica in use in the United States by mid-nineteenth century. The landmark works of Bigelow and of the Bartons (see C14 and C15) were out of print and "too expensive for general use," and according to the present work's author, C. Rafinesque's *Medical Flora* (see C17) contained "some important notices and facts on native plants but mingled with much that is incorrect and futile."

With emphasis on the botanical characters and classification of the medicinal plants, this book was intended as a companion to the more practical treatises, such as Wood and Bache's *United States Dispensatory* (see A4).

Arranged by botanical orders, and with over 300 illustrations, *Medical Botany* treats at length the most important articles of the vegetable materia medica, representing species from 123 orders and at least 400 genera. The monographs include, under the Latin names of the plants, the botanical descriptions, habitats, common names, physical descriptions, properties, medical uses, and how and by whom used. In most cases lengthy historical descriptions of the medical uses include doses of different dosage forms, comparison with other species of the same genus or of other genera, uses in other parts of the world, analyses of the plants, detection of adulteration, and preparations of the *United States Pharmacopoeia*. The book has an index of the common and foreign names of species and of vegetable products, and an index of orders, genera, and species, with their synonyms.

This single edition contains much information of phytochemical interest.

For a biographical sketch of this pioneer of American pharmacognosy, see B5.

C21 RUDOLPHY, John

> Chemical and pharmaceutical directory of all the chemicals and preparations (compound drugs) ... in general use in the drug trade. Their names and synonyms alphabetically arranged. In three parts: I English, Latin and German names; II Latin, German and English names; III German, Latin and English names. Chicago: John Rudolphy, 1877. 3 *l*, 8–407 p. 16×25 cm. (WU) **AIHP 67**

C22 RUDOLPHY, John

> Pharmaceutical directory of all the crude drugs now in general use; their etymology and names in alphabetical order. In four parts: I English, botanical,

pharmaceutical and German names; II Botanical, English, pharmaceutical and German names; III Pharmaceutical, botanical, English and German names; IV German, pharmaceutical, botanical and English names. Third edition. New York: William Radde, 1877. 8, 2 *l*, 5–119 p. 17×26 cm. (WU) **AIHP 68**

These two handbooks represent a singular type of pharmaceutical literature consisting of alphabetical lists of the names of medicinal substances; one handbook lists crude drugs and the other lists chemical and compound drugs. Both were intended as comprehensive references for druggists, physicians, and "the intelligent public in general."

The third (and final) enlarged and more comprehensive edition of the *Pharmaceutical Directory of Crude Drugs*, published originally in 1866, is presented here as a complement of the first edition of the *Chemical and Pharmaceutical Directory of Chemicals and Preparations*, both issued in the same year. The former is a compilation of the English, botanical, pharmaceutical, and German names of over 2000 crude drugs, arranged in four parts. Each part is an alphabetical list by one of the drug's names, with the other three names side by side following the primary entry.

The *Chemical and Pharmaceutical Directory of Chemicals and Preparations*, lists the English, Latin and German names "of all Compounds and preparations . . . in use by Druggists, Physicians and the Public in general," arranged in three parts. Each part is an alphabetical list by one of the names, with the other two names side by side. There are over 9,000 entries, including cross-references. A new revised edition was published in 1910 under the title *Pharmaceutical Directory and Handbook of All the Crude Drugs Now in General Use*. These works were compiled over many years by the Chicago druggist John Rudolphy.

C23 The modern materia medica. The source, chemical and physical properties, therapeutic action, dosage, antidotes and incompatibles of all additions to the newer materia medica that are likely to be called for on prescriptions. New York: The Druggists Circular, 1906. 2 *l*, 6–306 p. 12.5×18.5 cm. (WU) **AIHP 37**

This book exemplifies the dictionary-style of drug compendia of the early 1900s. It identifies "all the additions to the newer materia medica that are likely to be called for on Prescriptions," including "some older substances newly brought to the attention of the medical profession and ... a number of nutritives specially designed for use by the sick and convalescent." Published initially as an extended list in various issues of *The Druggists Circular, The Modern Materia Medica* is an alphabetical descriptive listing of over 2000 "new" remedies, whether of known or undisclosed composition, intended as a reference book for pharmacists. The entries vary in the extent of details: the information under each product may include synonyms, the source or the name of the person who introduced it, chemical and physical properties, use or therapeutic action, dose, dosage forms, precautions, antidotes, incompatibles, comparison with similar products, and trade names. Products of undisclosed composition are merely identified as such, sometimes indicating their active ingredients.

Other editions appeared in 1911 and 1912.

The commercial-technical journal from which this volume was collated was the first independent national journal of its kind in the United States. *The Druggists Circular* was published from 1857 to 1940 (until 1906 titled *The American Druggist's Circular and Chemical Gazette*).

Pharmacognosy

C24 MAISCH, John M[ichael], 1831–1893

A manual of organic materia medica. Being a guide to materia medica of the vegetable and animal kingdoms, for the use of students, druggists, pharmacists, and physicians. Philadelphia: Henry C. Lea's Son & Co., 1882. 1 *l*, iv–xv, 26–459 p. 13×19.5 cm. (ICRL) **AIHP 33**

One of the earliest American textbooks on materia medica adapted to pharmacy, this treatise pointed the way toward the study of scientific pharmacognosy, especially its chemical aspects, although definite steps in this direction had to wait for Power's translation of Flückiger and Tschirch's *Principles of Pharmacognosy* (see C25). The book introduced the author's own classification of drugs, which was similar to Flückiger's. Maisch's classification was based on the physical, histological, and chemical characteristics of drugs. Its purpose was to facilitate the recognition, determination of quality, and detection of adulteration of drugs, and the differentiation of their characteristic elements. Intended for students, druggists, pharmacists, and physicians, this manual won rapid acceptance. For many years its subsequent six editions were widely used, even though it had been preceded by a somewhat similar book of lesser scope, the *Conspectus of Organic Materia Medica and Pharmacal Botany*, by Lucius E. Sayre in 1879.

In three parts with over 190 illustrations, *A Manual of Organic Materia Medica* includes the drugs of the United States and British pharmacopoeias, and some important old and new unofficinal drugs. Part I covers animal drugs (e.g., eggs, calcareous skeletons, and secretions and excretions). Part II deals with cellular vegetable drugs, such as roots, barks, and flowers, and Part III with drugs without cellular structure, that is, extracts, sugars, resins, volatile oils, and so on. Each monograph, under the Latin name of the drug, includes the English name, origin, habitat, description, constituents, and properties and doses.

German-born John Michael Maisch emigrated to the United States in 1849, perhaps before obtaining any formal education. Diversely occupied in several cities, his scientific inclination led him to constant study and experimentation in chemistry as it related to pharmacy. In 1859 he began to teach in Parrish's School of Practical Pharmacy in Philadelphia, and two years later he was appointed to the chair of materia medica and pharmacy in the College of Pharmacy of the City of New York, at the same time he was employed in the laboratory of Edward R. Squibb. Maisch opened a drugstore in Philadelphia in 1865 and became active in the Philadelphia College of Pharmacy, as professor of pharmacy and materia medica in 1866, materia medica from 1867, and dean from 1879 until his death. One of the most important teachers, investigators, and writers on American pharmacy, his professional activities included: serving as editor of the *American Journal of Pharmacy*; holding several positions in the American Pharmaceutical Association, including service as its first permanent secretary from 1865 to 1893; playing a leading part in the revision of the *United States Pharmacopoeia*; and advocacy for the founding of state pharmaceutical associations and for state legislation declaring the duties and rights of the profession. Other publications include the third edition (1874) of R. Eglesfeld Griffith's *Universal Formulary* (see B5) and *Report on Legislation Regulating the Practice of Pharmacy in the United States* (see C40).

C25 FLÜCKIGER, Friedrich A., 1828–1894 and TSCHIRCH, Alexander, 1856–1939

The principles of pharmacognosy. An introduction to the study of the crude substances of the vegetable kingdom. Translated from the second ... revised German edition by Frederick B. Power. New York:

William Wood & Co., 1887. 1 *l*, iv–xvi, 294 p. 14.5×21.5 cm. (WU) **AIHP 18**

The work of Flückiger, from Switzerland, and of Tschirch, from Germany, together with Daniel Hanbury of England, laid the basis of modern pharmacognosy as a science. It was Tschirch who defined it as "the science the task of which is to recognize scientifically, to describe correctly and to arrange according to general principles, i.e., within a systematic order, the drugs of vegetable and animal origin taking into consideration all their peculiarities with the exception of their physiological effect."

Authors of various landmark works, Flückiger and Tschirch co-authored in 1885 the second edition of Flückiger's *Grundlagen der Pharmaceutischen Waarenkunde* ("Principles of Pharmaceutical Materia Medica," 1873). This book, with 186 illustrations, is presented here in an English translation by Frederick B. Power, who in view of the "generally acknowledged importance of the study of pharmacognosy," and of the reputation of the authors, wished that it "be made available to a larger circle of readers." Before the issuance of this American edition, John M. Maisch, influenced by the German literature, had ushered into American pharmacy the study of scientific pharmacognosy with his *Manual of Organic Materia Medica* (see C24), but it was *The Principles* that transmitted the full scientific conception.

Subtitled "An introduction to the study of the crude substances of the vegetable kingdom," the book was not intended as a complete text or manual; and its emphasis was not on specific drugs—these are mentioned only in connection with the morphology or anatomy of plants. Pointing to the relationship of pharmacognosy with chemical, botanical and microscopical science, the text is divided into seven major sections. An introduction on "The Mission of Pharmacognosy" is followed by "Treatment of the Subject Matter," which includes twelve topics, such as "The mother-plant," "Description of drugs," "Chemical constituents," and "Substitutions and adulterations." Next, "Aids to study" refers to collections and the literature, and "Morphology" covers eight plant parts, for example, roots, leaves, flowers, and seeds. The section on "Plant anatomy," the major portion of the book, deals in detail with the cell through systems of tissues. The last two sections are "Pathological formations" and "Microchemical reagents". It also has a thirteen-page index.

Only one edition was published.

A native of New York, Frederick Belding Power graduated from the Philadelphia College of Pharmacy in 1874, and two years later entered the University of Strassburg, receiving a Ph.D. degree in 1880. A pupil of Flückiger, he was appointed as his assistant.

Power held many prominent positions during his career and became well known for his plant chemistry research. He was professor and director of the chemical laboratory of the Philadelphia College of Pharmacy (1881–83), organizer and first director of the School of Pharmacy of the University of Wisconsin, and professor of materia medica and pharmacy (1883–92), scientific director of the Fritzsche Brothers Laboratories, where he conducted important research on essential oils (1892–96), director of the Henry S. Wellcome chemical research laboratories in London (1896–1914), and head of the Phytochemical Laboratory in the Bureau of Chemistry of the U.S. Department of Agriculture (1916). Among his many prizes and awards were the Ebert Prize on three occasions, and the Flückiger and Hanbury gold medals.

C26 KRAEMER, Henry, 1868–1924

Scientific and applied pharmacognosy. Intended for the use of students in pharmacy, as a handbook for pharmacists, and as a reference book for food and drug analysts and pharmacologists. Philadelphia: Published by the author, [c. 1915]. v–viii, 857 p. 15×22 cm. (WU) **AIHP 30**

Preceded by other pharmacognosy works of the late nineteenth century (see, for example, C24 and C25), this book, new in scope and presentation, was much used in the first half of the twentieth century. Characterizing pharmacognosy as an applied branch of botany and chemistry, it "abounds in illustrations which show that practical pharmacognosy is dependent upon the progress of scientific pharmacognosy." Based on many sources, mostly German and French, the book was intended for pharmacy students, as a handbook for pharmacists, and as a reference book for food and drug analysts and pharmacologists. Kraemer's *Applied and Economic Botany* (1915) supplemented this work with basic botanical facts and principles concerning medicinal and economic plants.

The drugs are arranged by families (about 100), with a summary of the morphological and histological characteristics of each family, with appropriate characterization and literature references for each drug. There are over 300 plates included among nearly 1000 illustrations. Some important animal drugs and a key for the identification of powdered drugs are also included. The book went through three editions until 1928. The third edition was the basis of *Pharmacognosy* by E. N. Gathercoal and E. H. Wirth (1936).

Henry Kraemer was professor of botany and pharmacognosy, and Director of the Microscopical Laboratory in the Philadelphia

College of Pharmacy when he compiled this book, positions that he held for twenty years (1897–1917). Born in Philadelphia, he served an apprenticeship of five years and graduated from the Philadelphia College of Pharmacy (Ph.G., 1889), from the School of Mines of Columbia University (Ph.B. in chemistry, 1895), and from the University of Marburg, Germany (Ph.D. in botany, 1896). He received an honorary Pharm.M. degree from the Philadelphia College of Pharmacy in 1928.

Kraemer's academic career included positions at the College of Pharmacy of the City of New York (1890), at the School of Pharmacy of Northwestern University (1896) and at the University of Michigan (1917–1920). Especially known for his research in botany and pharmacognosy, his other professional activities included editorship of the *American Journal of Pharmacy* for nearly twenty years (1898–1917), membership in the Committee of Revision of the United States Pharmacopoeia (1900) and in the Council on Pharmacy and Chemistry of the American Medical Association (1913–1921), and president of the American Conference of Pharmaceutical Faculties (1917).

Besides the book presented here, and the previously mentioned *Economic and Applied Botany*, Kraemer published *A Text Book of Botany and Pharmacognosy* (1902) that went through four editions to 1910, and was a collaborator in other scientific publications.

C27 YOUNGKEN, Heber W[ilkinson], 1885–1963

A text book of pharmacognosy. Philadelphia: P. Blakiston's Son & Co., [c. 1921]. 1 *l*, v–x, 1 *l*, 3–538 p. 15×23 cm. (DNLM) **AIHP 85**

Appearing when Kraemer's *Scientific and Applied Pharmacognosy* (see C26) was in its second edition and over twenty years after the final edition of Maisch's *A Manual of Organic Materia Medica* (see C24), this book became widely used. Going through six editions to 1948, it set the trend for more recent pharmacognosy textbooks. Its purpose was to serve as a textbook for students of pharmacognosy and as a reference book for drug analysts, pharmacognosists, wholesale and retail pharmacists, and crude drug collectors.

Based on the author's own research and a wide range of foreign and domestic publications, the book has 210 figures and 350 illustrations, and is arranged in two parts. Part I, "Morphologic Considerations of Drugs" (see C24) consists of Chapter I, "Fundamental Considerations" and Chapter II, "Morphological Classification of Crude Vegetable drugs," covering twenty-two forms, such as roots, rhizomes, bulbs, woods, and stems. Part II, "Taxonomic Considerations of Drugs" (see C26), consists also of two chapters: I "Crude Drugs of Vegetable Origin" (about ninety families), and II "Crude Drugs of Animal Origin" (six families). The book includes information such as synonyms, titles, habitats, physical characteristics and constituents of the crude drugs of U.S.P. IX and N.F. IV. In addition, many of the more common unofficial materials are included (such as unofficial drugs, condiments, spices, cereals, tea and chocolate), as well as drug adulterants, drug production and commerce, and descriptions of medicinal plants. A useful feature is a tabular comparison of commercial varieties of crude drugs and of drugs with their more common adulterants. The book has a two-page bibliography and an index.

Heber Wilkinson Youngken, a native of Pennsylvania, was professor of botany and pharmacognosy and Director of the Botanical Garden of the Philadelphia College of Pharmacy and Science when he wrote this book. He received degrees from the Medico-Chirurgical College of Philadelphia (Ph.G., 1905), Bucknell University (A.B., 1909), and the University of Pennsylvania (A.M., 1912, M.S., 1914, and Ph.D., 1915), and honorary degrees from the Philadelphia College of Pharmacy (Ph.M., 1919), Bucknell University (Sc.D., 1934), and the Massachusetts College of Pharmacy (Pharm.D., 1956).

After teaching in the Medico-Chirurgical College of Philadelphia, in the Philadelphia College of Pharmacy, and in Ursinus College, he was associated with the Massachusetts College of Pharmacy for four decades, from 1923 until his death, as professor in the Department of Materia Medica and as Emeritus Professor of Pharmacognosy and Botany (1957–63).

His professional activities included chairmanship of the Committee on Pharmacy, Botany and Pharmacognosy of the National Research Council for nearly twenty years (1923–42), membership in the U.S. Pharmacopoeial Convention (1920) and in many professional associations, including the American Pharmaceutical Association, where he was chairman of the Scientific Section (1921–22) and of the Historical Section (1935–36).

A recipient of the Ebert Prize on two occasions (1925 and 1931), Youngken's publications include *Pharmaceutical Botany* (seven editions from 1914 to 1951), and many papers and monographs. He was associate editor of the *United States Dispensatory* for the twenty-first to the twenty-fifth editions.

Pharmacology and Therapeutics

C28 SMITH, Peter, 1753–1816

The Indian doctor's dispensatory, being Father Smith's advice respecting diseases and their cure;

consisting of prescriptions for many complaints; and a description of medicines, simple and compound, showing their virtues and how to apply them. Designed for the benefit of children, his friends and the public, but more especially the citizens of the western parts of the United States of America. Cincinnati: Browne and Looker, Printers, 1813. i–iv, 108 p. 17.1×10 cm. (OCLloyd)

Representing a relatively large genre of American writings, *The Indian Doctor's Dispensatory* was a popular domestic medicine book, intended primarily for home doctoring by laymen, whereas the other works in this bibliography were meant primarily for use by medical and pharmaceutical practitioners. Actually the earliest American publications dealing significantly with the preparation and use of medicines were intended as much for self treatment by laymen as for practitioners of medicine and pharmacy, e.g., books such as Culpeper's *London Dispensatory* (see A1). Seemingly indispensable to the colonists, popular or domestic medicine books were quite common in the eighteenth and early nineteenth centuries. Comprehensive and practical, they sometimes included incidental advice for making simple remedies, and were occasionally designated as "dispensatories." The 1784 Philadelphia edition of *Domestic Medicine*, an early prototype of home doctoring books by William Buchan (a physician from Scotland) included what was called a "dispensatory."

A compilation of the author's own observations of fifty years, as well as information acquired from other physicians, *The Indian Doctor's Dispensatory* contains ninety prescriptions, mostly botanicals, which are "calculated to assist every citizen in the preservation of his health, and his recovery if diseased . . ." and reflect the idea that "the natives of our country are in possession of cures, simples, etc., that surpass what is used by our best practitioners."

These prescriptions are presented in numeric sequence under common names (no specific classification), in most cases with elaborate descriptions of the medicines and the uses of various simple forms of administration. Some prescriptions of mineral and animal products are included. The book also describes methods for artificial respiration, treatments of dislocated shoulders or broken bones, vaccine innoculation, and cold water applications. Prescriptions are given for such conditions as "dysentery," "ulcerated sore throat," "pleurisy," "inflammations and chronic pains," and "rising of a woman's breast."

As a student Peter Smith became familiar with such writers on "physic" as Culpeper (A1), B. S. Barton (C14), Samuel Thomson (C29) and William Brown (B1). Conversely, Rafinesque (C17) cited him as one of the authors consulted for his own book. A devout Baptist, Smith was a preacher, farmer, and practitioner of medicine who wandered through several states before finally settling in the Ohio country. Calling himself an "Indian doctor," he relied heavily on herbs, roots, and other remedies used by the Indians.

C29 THOMSON, Samuel, 1769–1843

New guide to health; or botanic family physician containing a complete system of practice, upon a plan entirely new; with a description of the vegetables made use of, and directions for preparing and administering them to cure disease. Boston: E. G. House, Printer, 1822. 2 *l*, 184–300 p., 1 *l*; bound together with an Introduction written by a friend. 10×17.5 cm. (WU) **AIHP 73**

Although there were several nineteenth-century botanico-medical sects, Thomsonianism was the first movement in the United States to defy regular medical and pharmaceutical practices. Founded on a system initiated by Samuel Thomson in the early 1800s, it rapidly won supporters; and when in 1813 Thomson was granted his first patent, it became the first and perhaps the only instance on record of a medical system being patented.

Before splitting up in 1838, the Thomsonians had boycotted regular drugstores, and developed their own pharmaceutical practice from infirmaries, depots and stores where botanic medicines were compounded and sold. Moreover, they were an effective force against medical licensing restrictions advocated by regular physicians.

Thomson published his *New Guide to Health* "to give a correct knowledge" of his system of medicine, from materials collected throughout thirty years of practice. Purchase of the book was tied to the purchase of the rights to use the system and to an agreement that "the purchasers, in consideration of . . . what is contained in this book, agree . . . not to reveal any part of said information to any person, except those who purchase the right."

The book contains some remarks on fevers and steaming, general directions for curing and preventing disease, descriptions of several cases of disease, and descriptions and directions for preparing and administering lobelia "to cleanse the stomach, overpower the cold, and promote free perspiration," and of capsicum "to retain vital heat."

After several enlarged and revised editions, the title of the book was changed to *The Thomsonian Materia Medica or Botanic Family*

Physician. A thirteenth edition was published in 1841, edited by the author's son John Thomson.

Born in New Hampshire of poor farming parents, Thomson at first worked as a farmer. Interested from an early age in the medicinal properties of plants, and convinced that he had a God-given gift for treating the sick, he eventually became a herbalist healer. With no education whatsoever, he was the founder of a botanico-medical sect bearing his name that exerted much medical and pharmaceutical influence during the first half of the nineteenth century.

C30 PAINE, Martyn, 1794–1877

Essays on the philosophy of vitality . . . and on the modus operandi of remedial agents. New York: Hopkins & Jennings, Printer, 1842. 2 *l*, v–viii, 2–70 p. 14.5×22.5 cm. (DNLM) **AIHP 46**

This book is an early attempt by an American physician to explain drug action in terms of the altered properties of the vital principle. It was written "to counteract the influence of the iatro-chemical philosophers," in view of "the tendency of the labours now in progress in organic chemistry to the subversion of physiological science, and therefore of pathological and therapeutic principle." An earlier somewhat similar work, but of no discernible influence, was an M.D. thesis written by William Wyatt Bibb in 1801 (*An Inquiry into the Modus Operandi of Medicines upon the Human Body*, Philadelphia, 68 p.).

The book consists of two parts, each one about thirty-five pages. The first part, "Essays on Vitality as Contra-Distinguished from Chemical and Mechanical Philosophy," is an argumentation in favor of "the vital principle" supported by excerpts from the works of therapists such as Frenchmen Xavier Bichat and Gabriel Andral. Its prime contention is that "an attempt to overthrow the experience of the past . . . by a distorted construction of 'facts' which are yielded by test glasses and crucibles, appears . . . to be an enterprise which should alarm physiologists as to its pernicious consequences." In the second part, "On the Modus Operandi of Remedial Agents," also reinforced by Bichat and Andral, it is argued that the action of medicines is based on the restoration of the altered forces or properties of the vital principle, and that the "partial absorption of certain remedies is only a contingent result and has little or no agency in the physiological phenomena."

For a biographical sketch of Martyn Paine, see C19.

C31 HERING, C[onstantin], 1800–1880

Condensed materia medica, compiled with the assistance of Drs. A. Korndoerfer and E. A. Farrington. New York and Philadelphia: Boericke and Tafel, 1877. 1 *l*, vii–xvi, 870 p., 1 *l*. 16×22 cm. (WU) **AIHP 23**

Written by a founder of homeopathy in the United States, this book foreshadows the author's most significant work, the ten-volume *Guiding Symptoms*, published at a later date (1879–1896). Intended as a manual for students and practitioners of homeopathy, it contains essential material on the leading symptoms and characteristics of each remedy. Although limited to only 184 remedies out of thousands recognized for use, it is comprehensive in the presentation of drug-induced symptoms and illustrates adequately the homeopathic utility of each remedy.

The remedies are presented in alphabetical sequence by Latin names. The symptoms produced by the remedies, as the basis of homeopathic therapeutics, are given under forty-eight divisions (chapters). For example, the symptoms "very dull," and "low spirited" appear under the chapter entitled "mind and disposition," which concerns all mental states, and the symptom "vertigo" is listed under the chapter heading "sensorium," which embraces oversensitiveness and irritability of the brain and senses.

Born in Germany, Constantin Hering received a medical degree from the University of Wurzburg in 1826. Nine years later he arrived in Philadelphia where he practiced medicine until his death. He was co-founder of the first American homeopathic college, the North American Academy of the Homoeopathic Art, in 1835; of the American Institute of Homeopathy, this country's first national medical society, in 1844; and of the Homeopathic College of Pennsylvania in 1848, becoming professor of materia medica, and dean when it merged with the Hahnemann Medical College in 1871. He established the *American Journal of Homoeopathic Materia Medica*, wrote more than 300 articles, mostly on remedies with indications for their use, and edited or wrote nearly ninety books and pamphlets.

C32 CUSHNY, Arthur Robertson, 1866–1926

A textbook of pharmacology and therapeutics or the action of drugs in health and disease. Philadelphia and New York: Lea Brothers & Co., 1899. 2 *l*, 6–730 p. 14.5×23 cm. (ICRL) **AIHP 10**

Based on experimental laboratory work, this book is often considered the first modern text of pharmacology in the English language. For medical students beginning their clinical studies, it intended "to show how far the clinical effects of remedies may be explained by their action on the normal body, and how these may be in turn correlated with physiological phenomena."

The author relied on numerous major original papers, French and German textbooks, his own experimentation, and was markedly influenced by Oswald Schmiedeberg's classical *Grundriss der Arzneimittellehre.*

The book examines mostly the medicinal preparations recognized by the United States and British pharmacopoeias, but also includes unimportant drugs because "the teacher of pharmacology must not only point out the good, but has the more ungrateful task of condemning the worthless." Illustrated with forty-seven engravings, the book is divided into six parts with a twenty-three-page introduction that briefly covers the following topics: the mode of action of drugs, stimulation, depression and irritation, elective affinity of drugs and protoplasm poisons, chemical composition and pharmacological action, conditions modifying the effects of drugs, methods of administration, pharmacopoeias and pharmacopoeial preparations, and classification of drugs. Part I deals with organic substances used for their local action; Part II (the most extensive part) covers thirty-two topics in 339 pages dealing with organic substances used for their action after absorption; Part III covers combinations of the alkalies, alkaline earths, acids and allied bodies; Part IV deals with the heavy metals, Part V with ferments, secretions and toxalbumins, and Part VI with menstrua and mechanical remedies.

By 1937 this text had been through at least eleven editions and was the second most widely used text in schools of pharmacy, after Sollman's *A Manual of Pharmacology* (see C34).

Arthur Robertson Cushny, M.A. and M.D., was a native of Scotland. After studies in Aberdeen and Berne, he learned the elements of physiological technique from Schmiedeberg at Strassburg, and was his assistant in 1892–1893. A professor of pharmacology and therapeutics for over thirty years, he taught at the University of Michigan (1893–1905), at the University College, London (1905–1918), and in the University of Edinburgh (1918–1926). His investigations on the effects of digitalis, and his controlled experiments on the mammalian heart were renowned. Other subjects with which he is prominently identified are the contrasted action of optical isomers and the mechanism of urinary secretion.

C33 New and non-official remedies. A reprint from the *Journal of the American Medical Association* of the articles tentatively approved by the Council on Pharmacy and Chemistry of the American Medical Association. Chicago:

Press of the American Medical Association, March 30, 1907. 1 *l*, 4–112 p. 13×21 cm. (WU) **AIHP 42**

This annual publication was important for at least fifty years as one of the best known examples of American authoritative books supplementary to the official drug standards of the United States. First published serially in the *Journal of the American Medical Association*, this first edition is a selective compilation reporting on more than 1500 proprietary products of disclosed composition that were approved by the Council on Pharmacy and Chemistry of the American Medical Association. Approval of these products—according to a set of rules applicable to the medicaments and to their advertising, naming, labeling, and policies of the manufacturers—was based on evidence submitted by the manufacturers and on investigations made or directed by the Council. Admission of a product to "NNR" did not necessarily imply a recommendation, but came to be regarded as a sign of impending official acceptance or of the recognition of the product by the medical profession as a respectable part of the drug therapy.

Following the rules of approval, the monographs appear in alphabetical order and include at least the following information: title, concentration of active ingredients or pharmaceutical formula, definition or description (including, for chemicals, tests for identity, purity and strength, and structural formulas, if known), actions and uses, dosage in the decimal and apothecary systems, manufacturer, place of registration, and patent numbers.

The title changed to *New and Non-Official Drugs* in 1958, then to *New Drugs Evaluated by the A.M.A. Council on Drugs*, of which three editions were published from 1965 to 1967.

The Council was organized in 1905 mainly to gather and diffuse "such information as would protect the medical profession in the prescribing of proprietary medicinal articles." Renamed Council on Drugs in 1958, it was abolished in 1972, reflecting changes occuring in the drug market and in the Association.

C34 SOLLMAN, Torald, 1874–1965

A manual of pharmacology and its applications to therapeutics and toxicology. Philadelphia and London: W.B. Saunders Company, 1917. 1 *l*, 9–901 p. 16×23.5 cm. (WU)

Arthur Cushny's *A Textbook of Pharmacology and Therapeutics* (see C32) was in its second edition when Torald Sollman published the *Text-Book of Pharmacology and Some Allied Sciences*

(1901). After subsequent rearrangement and enlargement this textbook became the *Manual*, a quite different book. Intended as a text and reference book, it put together the essentials of pharmacology, detailed data for consultation, and bibliographic references. About twenty years later, the fourth edition of this book (1932) was the most widely used textbook in American schools of pharmacy, surpassing Cushny's work (Eleventh Edition, 1936) (see C32).

The text is organized under about 170 diverse topics, some treated briefly, others considered in more detail and divided into subtopics. To illustrate, the first eighty pages cover twelve subjects, of which "Classes of Pharmaceutic Preparations" and "The Treatment of Disease" comprise about half the contents. Other subjects treated briefly include pharmacognosy, important plant constituents, general toxicology, prescription writing, and coloring and flavoring. Some headings in the rest of the text refer to drug action or effect. For example, ferments and nutrients, emollients, phenomena common to local irritants, corrosives and astringents, non-volatile organic irritants, drugs employed for their local effects on the alimentary canal, the cocaine group, local anesthetics, drugs acting peripherally on the autonomic-sympathetic system, and pharmacology of heat regulation. Most of the contents, however, appear under the names of the drugs. The information under each drug includes action and uses, preparations, absorption, fate, excretion, and systemic action.

The essentials of pharmacology as of 1917 appear in large print, while detailed and documented data for consultation are given in small print.

Three appendices contain a tabulation of average doses, a checklist of important preparations, and a sixty-two-page bibliography.

The book went through eight editions to 1957.

German-born Torald Hermann Sollman studied chemistry in Paris (1893–94) and received an M.D. degree from Western Reserve University Medical School in 1896. Associated with this institution for nearly seven decades, he occupied academic positions from 1895 to 1965, first as demonstrator in physiology, then as professor of pharmacology and materia medica, dean (1928–44), and emeritus professor (1944–65).

Prominent in professional activities, he was a founding member of the American Society for Pharmacology and Experimental Therapeutics and of the American Medical Association's Council on Pharmacy and Chemistry, and a member of the Committee of Revision of the *United States Pharmacopoeia* (1910–1930). His widely-used textbooks and laboratory manuals are excellent mirrors of the state of pharmacology in their time.

Pharmaceutical Chemistry

C35 BECK, Lewis C[aleb], 1798–1853

Adulteration of various substances used in medicine and the arts with the means of detecting them. New York: Samuel S. and William Wood, 1846. xi, 332 p. 12.5×20 cm. (DNLM) **AIHP 04**

The problem of drug adulteration, known since at least the first century A.D., was dealt with in antiquity through crude and primarily sensorial tests for the identity and quality of drugs. It was not until the late eighteenth and early nineteenth centuries, after refinement of the microscope and the emergence of modern analytical chemistry, that scientific methods began to be devised. These developments were reflected for the first time in the United States in U.S.P. II (1842), with the introduction of simple tests for specific gravity and solubility, and qualitative tests for determining the authenticity and purity of some simple and compound drugs. By this time adulteration ordinarily meant contamination of a drug, with the effect of weakening its medicinal power, and the average drug dispenser was poorly equipped to detect it.

The book presented here, the only edition of the earliest American treatise that included the detection of drug adulteration, was opportune in a time of frequent drug deceit. This problem had prompted earlier the foundation of the first local associations (colleges) of pharmacy, and later of the first national pharmaceutical association (American Pharmaceutical Association, 1852), and the enactment of the first federal drug import law (1848).

Intended as a manual for physicians, pharmacists, and artisans, it gives simple processes for the qualitative and in some cases, roughly quantitative detection of adulteration. Its sources were some current foreign texts on applied analytical chemistry, food adulteration, and materia medica, and American works such as the *United States Dispensatory*. Arranged alphabetically by English names, the manual describes about 270 substances in the pure state, with their synonyms, the U.S.P. names for medicinals, and procedures for the detection of possible adulterants. A three-part appendix describes the operations and instruments of qualitative analysis and the preparation of reagents; and five tables give the behavior of some reagents with the more important metals, metallic oxides and acids.

A book on a similar topic, adapted to the 1848 drug import law, was written some years later by an examiner of medicines for the port of Boston: C. H. Peirce, *Examination of Drugs, Medicines,*

Chemicals, Etc., as to Their Purity and Adulterations (Cambridge, Mass, 1852). One other edition was published the next year.

Physician Lewis Caleb Beck issued his book while professor of chemistry at Rutgers College in New Jersey and at the Albany Medical College in New York State. A native of New York, he received his education in that state, and practiced medicine there before turning to education and research. He authored over twenty books on medicine, chemistry, botany, and mineralogy, and contributed to the detection of purity of foods and drugs.

C36 ATTFIELD, John, 1835–1911

Chemistry: general, medical and pharmaceutical. Philadelphia: Henry C. Lea, 1871. iii–xi, 14–552 p. 11.5×18.5 cm. (WU) **AIHP 01**

During the mid-nineteenth century, American pharmacy derived its learning in chemistry from British texts or American editions of them. Of lasting popularity over a period of at least thirty years were the nine American editions of Attfield's *Chemistry: General, Medical, and Pharmaceutical*. The first American edition (from the second London edition, 1869) is presented here.

Intended for students and practitioners of medicine and of pharmacy, this book was designed as a practical handbook and reference manual and as a reading book for those unable to attend lectures or perform experiments. Two features, at least, distinguished it from other contemporary texts: the omission of material interesting only to the scientific chemist, and the inclusion of the chemistry of the preparations and the materia medica of the *United States Pharmacopoeia* (Fourth Revision 1863, reprinted 1864, 1866, 1868). Other traits are: repeated consideration of the same facts or principles from different chemical viewpoints (i.e., physical, synthetical, analytical, or quantitative), explanation of general difficulties, such as nomenclature, notation and chemical constitution as they appear, rather than in introductory chapters or general remarks, and the addition of study questions under each subject.

Attfield's *Chemistry* is divided into nineteen thematic sections. An introductory review of the principal properties of the elements is followed by the general principles of chemical theory, a detailed description of the metallic and non-metallic compounds and their officinal preparations and tests, systematic analysis, the chemistry of some natural products, and practical toxicology, and the chemical and microscopical characters of morbid urine, urinary sediment, and calculi. The final sections form a laboratory guide for chemical and physical quantitative analysis. The appendix includes a table of tests for impurities in preparations of the *British Pharmacopoeia*, tables of saturation of acids and alkalies designed for use in prescribing and dispensing, a table of strength of alcoholic liquids, and the elements with their symbols and atomic weights.

Attfield's book was promptly accepted over George Fownes's *Elementary Chemistry, Theoretical and Practical* (Philadelphia, 1845), a British text of which the first American edition had appeared about three decades earlier, with successive editions published until 1878. In the 1850s Fownes's work was preferred to others because of its clearness and conciseness, but later editions became more comprehensive and difficult.

Pharmacy-educator John Attfield, Ph.D., served as director and professor of practical chemistry for the Pharmaceutical Society of Great Britain for over thirty years (1862–1896). Exerting a profound influence, he has been considered a "father of modern English pharmacy." He was an honorary member of the colleges of pharmacy of Philadelphia, New York, and Chicago.

C37 HOFFMANN, Frederick, 1832–1904

Manual of chemical analysis as applied to the examination of medicinal chemicals. A guide for the determination of their identity and quality, and for the detection of impurities and adulterations. For the use of pharmaceutists, physicians, druggists, and manufacturing chemists and of pharmaceutical and medical students. New York: D. Appleton & Co., 1873. 1 *l*, iii, 8–393 p. 14.5×22.5 cm. (ICRL) **AIHP 25**

This book, the earliest chemical text written in the United States by a pharmacist, was the first one focusing solely on the determination of identity and quality, and on the detection of impurities and adulterations of medicinal chemicals. For the use of pharmaceutists, physicians, druggists, manufacturing chemists, and pharmaceutical and medical students, it was intended as a ready reference guide in the application of essentially qualitative chemical analysis to drug analysis.

Although numerous current books and periodicals were consulted and used freely, none were listed because it "would have greatly increased the size of the volume, without offering a corresponding advantage."

Compiled with special reference to the *United States Pharmacopoeia* (Fifth Revision, 1873), the *British Pharmacopoeia* (Second Revision, 1867), and the *Pharmacopoea Germanica* of 1872, the subject matter is arranged in two parts. The first part serves as a preliminary background, containing some remarks on manipulations and reagents and on a few important general tests, and a brief outline for the systematic qualitative analysis and volumetric estimation of medicinal chemicals. The second part, the greater component of the book (over 300 pages), describes the physical and chemical properties of about 200 compounds (mostly inorganic) and their preparations, and the methods for determining their identity, quality and purity. The arrangement is alphabetical by Latin names. The absence of chemical notation to express the constitution of the compounds is noteworthy.

A second edition of the book (1883) was co-authored by Frederick B. Power.

German-born Frederick Hoffmann, Ph.D., greatly influenced early American pharmacy during more than thirty years of pharmaceutical activity as a pharmacist, editor, and analytical chemist. He was active in the approval of the first pharmacy laws of New York in 1872, and in the compilation of the Sixth Revision of the *United States Pharmacopoeia* in 1880, which became the modern model for future revisions. He founded the *Pharmaceutische Rundschau* in 1882, which was published in German until 1896, when it became the English language *Pharmaceutical Review*.

C38 LYONS, A[lbert] B[rown], 1841–1926

Manual of practical pharmaceutical assaying, including details of the simplest and best methods of determining the strength of crude drugs and of galenical preparations. Designed especially for the use of the student and of the practical pharmacist. Detroit: D. O. Haynes & co., 1886. iii–vi, 7–154 p. 12.5×17 cm. (WU) **AIHP 31**

This is the first book issued in the United States dealing exclusively with pharmaceutical assaying, particularly alkaloidal standardization. The work put into it marked the beginning of a major development in American pharmacy: the production of uniform medicinal preparations. Covering only about thirty assays, it might seem limited in scope; however, "They are offered for what they are worth, in the belief that to those who do not read German they will be of material service, and that from that small beginning there will soon arise . . . a literature in our own tongue of a subject of such growing importance." These assays were essentially developed by the author, but his sources included the German work of Professor Georg Dragendorff, one of the most prominent pharmacists of his time, and the contributions of the well-known pharmaceutical manufacturer, Edward R. Squibb.

Designed for the student and the pharmacist, the book contains simple methods for determining the strength, in terms of active constituents, of crude drugs and their preparations. With illustrations and diagrams, and with many bibliographic footnotes, the text is arranged under about forty captions, including general topics such as apparatus required, reagents, general methods of assay of crude drugs, methods of extracting alkaloids from crude drugs, gravimetric estimation of alkaloids, assay of galenical preparations and estimation of alcohol and glycerin in fluid extracts. Also, assay methods for specific drugs and their preparations were included in alphabetical sequence, for example, aconite, cinchona bark, digitalis, hydrastis, and podophyllum. An appendix consists of a tabulation of results of assays of some of the more important drugs.

Revision of the *Manual* resulted in a new book by the same author, *Handbook of Practical Assaying of Drugs and Galenicals* (1899), which in turn was replaced by another entirely new text, *Practical Standardization by Chemical Assay of Organic Drugs and Galenicals* (Detroit, 1920, 397 p.). The latter is a much enlarged and rearranged volume, written after the author's retirement, for pharmacy students and practicing pharmacists, but also for the manufacturer, the control chemist, and the drug inspector. It consists of two parts: one of general principles and procedures and another of methods of assay and standardization of individual drugs.

Born in Hawaii, Albert Brown Lyons received his early education at Oahu College and an M.D. degree from the University of Michigan in 1868. Having also studied pharmaceutical chemistry (under A. B. Prescott), he became assistant and then professor of chemistry at Detroit College of Medicine, a position he held for twelve years, while at the same time operating a pharmacy. Discontinuing his nexus with teaching and the practice of pharmacy, from 1881 to 1888 he was an analytical and consulting chemist at Parke, Davis and Company. There he pioneered the standardization of pharmaceutical preparations, particularly fluid extracts of alkaloidal drugs, and wrote the book presented here. As a founder of alkaloidal assaying in the United States, his leadership in this field showed the way for succeeding research scientists—perhaps his most significant contribution to pharmacy and medicine.

An active member of the American Pharmaceutical Association, he was elected honorary president in 1915. The first editor of *Pharmaceutical Era* (1887) and author of *Plant Names, Scientific and Popular* (1890), he had a wide reputation as an authority on botanical nomenclature and synonyms.

C39 PITTENGER, Paul S., b. 1889

Biochemic drug assay methods with special reference to the pharmacodynamic standardization of

drugs. Philadelphia: P. Blakiston's Son & Co., [c. 1914].
1 *l*, v–xv, 158 p. 13.5×17.5 cm. (WU) **AIHP 61**

This is the first American text on the biostandardization of drugs. Intended as a manual "for students of pharmacy, pharmaceutic chemistry and medicine," and for use by pharmacists and pharmaceutical chemists in drug standardization laboratories, it introduced the concept that the purpose of pharmacodynamic assaying was to secure preparations of uniform therapeutic activity, not to determine the real value of a drug in the treatment of disease.

Using monographs, government bulletins, papers read before medical and pharmaceutical societies, and especially the author's own research observations as sources, the book explains in a clear narrative style the most widely-used methods and apparatus then current. Eighty-nine pictures and diagrams illustrate the eight chapters. The chapter topics are "Preliminary Considerations," "Cardiac Stimulants and Depressants," "Epinephrine and Products of the Suprarenal Gland," "Ergot," "Pituitary Extracts," "Cannabis Indica," "Technique and Apparatus Employed," and "Solutions."

When Paul A. Pittenger prepared this book he was instructor in pharmacodynamics at the Medico-Chirurgical College of Philadelphia. There the well-known professor of materia medica and botany, physician and pharmacy graduate Francis E. Stewart (1853–1941) collaborated with him in preparing the text. A native of Easton, Pennsylvania, Pittenger received degrees from the Medico-Chirurgical College (Pharmacy 1909, Pharmaceutical Chemistry 1910, and Pharmacodynamics, 1911) and from the Philadelphia College of Pharmacy (Ph.M. 1919, and an Sc.D. 1940 for distinguished service in the standardization of drugs).

As a teacher and author he was of prime importance in the early development of drug bioassay; as Director of Pharmacodynamic Research at the H. K. Mulford Company (1910–1925) he guided the company to a position of early leadership in biological drug standardization. He was a member of several professional and scientific societies and committees, including the Committee of Revision of the U.S.P. X, and the Committee on Physiological Testing of the American Pharmaceutical Association, which he chaired for eleven years (1918–1929). Contributing frequently to the scientific literature, he wrote one other book on biological standardization: *A Textbook of Biologic Assay* (Philadelphia, 1928).

Laws and Regulations

C40 MAISCH, John M., 1831–1893

Report on legislation regulating the practice of pharmacy in the United States. Philadelphia: Merrihew and Son, Printers, 1868. 48 p. 14×22.5 cm. (WU) **AIHP 32**

This pamphlet represents the first effort in the United States to compile and review the existing or projected laws or parts of laws related to pharmacy. It is reprinted in the 1868 *Proceedings of the American Pharmaceutical Association* (Philadelphia, 1869), pp. 329–370. Concern for the status of "state laws for the protection of the interests of the profession of Pharmacy, for the suppressing of empyricism" was expressed as early as the 1852 founding meeting of the American Pharmaceutical Association. About sixteen years later, John M. Maisch, the permanent secretary of the Association and author of this pamphlet, requested from state authorities and association members in each state copies of enacted or planned state laws bearing upon the practice of pharmacy, the education of pharmacists, and the required qualifications for practice; and information on the operation of these laws and their effect on the public and on the medical and pharmaceutical professions.

The *Report* presented here lists the seventeen states and one territory that responded to the inquiry, including the states of Alabama, Florida, Georgia, Massachusetts, Minnesota, Wisconsin, and eleven others, and the territory of New Mexico. Only Georgia responded that it had state regulations intending to limit the practice of pharmacy to competent persons as part of the Code of the State of Georgia (1867). Pennsylvania and New York reported that they had only local laws; these were reprinted and commented on in the *Report*, as well as the Georgia regulations. Also included in it are sections of existing laws pertaining to other important issues of American pharmacy in the 1860s, such as counter-prescribing, quackery, secret remedies, the sale of intoxicating liquors, abortifacients, and poisons, the adulteration of drugs and medicines, and the formation of associations.

When the report was read before the sixteenth annual meeting of the Association (1868), a resolution was approved to send copies of the *Report* "to the libraries of the several State legislatures, to the Governors of several States, and the leading Judges of the Courts." The report became the precursor of a "draft of a proposal to regulate the practice of pharmacy and the sale of poisons and to prevent adulteration of drugs and medicines," prepared by John M. Maisch and a special committee, and presented at the next annual meeting (1869). Despite not having the Association's formal approval, this proposal was distributed to the legislatures and governors of each state, and became the basis of the first state pharmacy laws in this country.

For a biographical sketch of John M. Maisch, see C24.

C41 Wedderburn, Alex J.

A compilation of the pharmacy and drug laws of the several states and territories. U.S. Department

of Agriculture, Division of Chemistry, Bulletin No.
42. Washington, D.C.: Government Printing Office, 1894.
1 *l*, 3–152 p. 14.5×22.5 cm. (WU) **AIHP 77**

This government pamphlet is a compilation of the forty-three
acts regulating the practice of pharmacy and the dispensing of drugs,
medicines, poisons, or intoxicating liquors that were in force in the
United States as of June 1893. They are either pharmacy laws that
include sections on drugs, or individual pharmacy laws and drug
laws enacted separately, or pharmaceutical sections of general statutes. Based on information supplied by officers of the state pharmaceutical associations, there were no laws in the states of Indiana,
Maryland (except for Baltimore), Montana and Nevada, or in the
Indian Territory and the territory of Arizona. According to the com-
piler, there was no pharmacy or drug law in Idaho, although *Kremers
and Urdang's History of Pharmacy* (Fourth Edition) lists an 1887
territorial law.

Alex J. Wedderburn was a special agent in the U.S. Department of Agriculture when he compiled these laws.

Another publication of the same year, limited to the New England laws, was *The Law of the Apothecary* by George H. Fall, a
compendium for "apothecaries and chemists." While Wedderburn's
pamphlet is solely a compilation of laws, Fall gives, besides the text
of the laws, an explanation of their principles in common language.

C42 WILEY, Harley R., d. 1924

A treatise on pharmacal jurisprudence with a thesis
on the law in general. San Francisco: The Hicks-Judd
Co., 1904. 3 *l*, 4–262 p. 12.5×19.5 cm. (WU) **AIHP 80**

This book defining the principles of the legal aspects of the
profession of pharmacy in the United States was issued because of
the "inconvenience experienced through the want of some treatise,
or collection of authorities on pharmacal law." Intended as a textbook for a pioneer course in pharmaceutical law at the University
of California, it explains the substance of the law and cites a na-
tionwide selection of 190 illustrative cases, which are listed alphabetically at the beginning of the book with page locations.

An introduction, on the law in general, deals with the beginnings of law, the American system of jurisprudence, federal, state,
supreme law, and international law, comity between the states, and
equity. In a narrative style, seventeen chapters cover numerous subjects under such general headings as "Legal Limits of Pharmacy,"
"The Common Law Right to Practice Pharmacy, and the Reason

for Statutory Restriction on the Right," "Contracts of Druggists and Pharmacists," "Liability for Error in Preparing Prescriptions," "Liability of the Manufacturing Pharmacist," and "The Pharmacist in Court." A useful feature is a detailed outlined index.

Only one edition was published.

A graduate of Trinity College (1877), Harley R. Wiley was for some time principal of schools in Redding, California, and in 1883 conducted California's first normal institute. He graduated from the University of California law department in 1891, and was lecturer on pharmaceutical law in the College of Pharmacy for twenty-five years, lecturing also at the College of Sciences and the College of Dentistry. *A Treatise* grew out of his lectures at the College of Pharmacy.

C43 KEBLER, Lyman F., 1863–1955

Drug legislation in the United States revised to July 15, 1908. U.S. Department of Agriculture, Bureau of Chemistry Bulletin No. 98 (revised). Part I. Washington, D.C.: Government Printing Office, 1909. 2–343 p. 14.5×23 cm. (WU) **AIHP 27**

Compiled in the Division of Drugs of the United States Department of Agriculture Bureau of Chemistry, this bulletin was intended as a reference for legislators, physicians, pharmacists, and government officials. Depicting drug control measures in the early twentieth century, it was an update of a 1906 compilation including "all existing laws . . . enacted for the purpose of minimizing the sale of adulterated and deteriorated drugs and for safeguarding the public health by restricting the sale of poisonous and habit-forming drugs." Although intended as a two-part publication, apparently Part II was never published.

This publication contains the 1906 Federal Food and Drug Act and sections of the 1848 federal drug import law, and other federal laws dealing with such topics as the dispensing of alcoholic medicinal compounds and antitoxic serums, the importation of opium, and the sale of abortifacients. It also summarizes the drug laws in all the states (forty-six) and territories (six), and in the District of Columbia. There are also sections pertaining to the role of pharmacists, the sale of poisons, the adulteration and misbranding of drugs, and the itinerant vending of drugs.

The historical value of this document as a primary source is enhanced by a background note on the conditions prior to the 1848 federal drug import law, quoting from a Congressional report, and by references indicating where the laws were found as they appear in the compilation ("general" references) and as originally enacted ("historical" references).

Pharmaceutical chemist and physician Lyman F. Kebler was Chief of the Division of Drugs of the U.S.D.A. Bureau of Chemistry when he compiled the bulletin introduced here, a position he held for sixteen years (1907–1923). A native of Michigan, he graduated from the University of Michigan (Ph.C. 1890, B.S. 1891, M.S. 1892) and from George Washington University (M.D. 1906). In industry, government, and academic positions for at least four decades, he made contributions on chemical, nutritional, and medical subjects. He was a member of the Committee of Revision of the *United States Pharmacopoeia* (1910–1920) and secretary of the Pharmacopoeial Convention from 1920 to 1930. His membership in professional associations included the American Chemical Society, the American Medical Association, and the American Pharmaceutical Association; in the latter he was chairman of the Scientific Section (1901–02) and of the Historical Section (1928–29).

C44 WILBERT, Martin I., 1865–1916 and MOTTER, Murray Galt, 1866–1926

Digest of laws and regulations in force in the United States relating to the possession, use, sale, and manufacture of poisons and habit-forming drugs. United States Public Health Service, Public Health Bulletin No. 56. Washington, D.C.: Government Printing Office, 1912. 1 *l*, 3–278 p. 15×23 cm. (WU) **AIHP 79**

Differing from Kebler's *Drug Legislation* (see C43) in scope, intent and format, this bulletin facilitates a comparison of the legal requirements pertaining to poisons and habit-forming drugs in the United States and its territories as of July 1912. Prepared by order of the Surgeon General, *Digest of Laws* includes an alphabetical list by geographical areas of the legal codes and other authorities consulted. In addition there are six comparative tables on topics such as the number of suicides and deaths from acute and chronic poisoning and alcoholism (1900–1910), requirements to restrict the sale of poisons and the sale and use of cocaine and narcotics, and requirements relating to the practice of pharmacy in the laws regulating the sale of poisons and narcotics, and two lists: one of general definitions and the other of substances enumerated in the laws to restrict the sale of poisons.

The major portion of the volume consists of excerpts and references to all current federal, state and territorial laws, and to municipal ordinances, rules and regulations of cities with a population over 25,000. For the United States (federal) and for each state and territory, these excerpts are presented under the following headings: "Sale and use of poisons," "Sale and use of cocaine and narcotics," "Drugs to be announced on label," "Poisons in articles of commerce," "Occupational intoxications," "Methyl alcohol," "Practice of pharmacy," "Standards for drugs," and "Sale and use of intoxicating liquors." Under the last-mentioned heading are included only laws recognizing alcohol as a poison and a narcotic, and relating to the sale of alcohol, and of alcohol-containing beverages by pharmacists. A useful feature of this book is an index organized so that in effect it is a comparative summary of the legislation cited.

The authors prepared this digest while associated with the United States Public Health Service. Pharmacist Wilbert was an assistant in the Division of Pharmacology of the Hygienic Laboratory (1908–1916), and physician Motter, a professor of physiology at Georgetown University and active in Pharmacopoeial work, was director of USPHS library services.

Born in New York, Martin I. Wilbert graduated from the Philadelphia College of Pharmacy in 1890 and received a master of pharmacy degree from the same institution thirteen years later (1903). As chief apothecary of the German Hospital of Philadelphia for seventeen years, he became an ingenious pioneer in American hospital pharmacy. He was an active member of the American Pharmaceutical Association and of the American Medical Association, belonging to the latter's Council on Pharmacy and Chemistry. A member of the revision committees for U.S.P. IX and N.F. IV, his *Digest of Comments* on these works received favorable reviews. A prolific writer, his works included many pharmaco-historical articles.

C45 O'CONNELL, C. Leonard, 1890–1958 and PETTIT, William, 1907–1982

A manual on pharmaceutical law. Together with appendices containing important laws of Congress, the uniform narcotic drug law, and other laws relating to pharmacy. Philadelphia: Lea Febiger, 1938. 2 *l*, 6–196 p. 13.5×20 cm. (WU) **AIHP 43**

Published over three decades after Wiley's *Treatise* (see C42), this book exemplifies texts on pharmaceutical law intended for American pharmacy students and practicing pharmacists in the late 1930s. Analyzing and comparing state laws, summarizing legal decisions and comments, and providing the full text of important laws,

Pharmaceutical Law is a useful historical source on regulation of drugs and pharmacy practice during that period.

In eight chapters, the book covers over thirty topics, for example, police power, state boards of pharmacy, qualifications of applicants, state pure drug laws, Federal Pure Food and Drugs Act, Federal Trade Commission Act, the handling of unusual-quantity prescriptions, duty as to maintenance of a drug store, negligence in selling, clerk's authority to bind owner in contract, ownership of prescription, pharmacist practicing medicine, warranties in sales of drugs, price-fixing agreements, basis and purpose of bankruptcy law, and insurance protection for pharmacists. It includes a comparative table of the requirements for entrance to state board examinations in all the states and territories, three appendices, and a subject index. The appendices are: I Important Federal Laws, II Uniform Narcotic Drug Act, and III Pennsylvania Laws of Pharmacy.

Co-author William Pettit, a member of the Pittsburgh Bar and later lecturer in pharmaceutical jurisprudence at the University of Pittsburgh, issued under the same title an updated book similar to this one in scope and format (New York, 1949), of which a second edition appeared in 1957 and a third in 1962 (reprinted in 1965 and 1970).

Charles Leonard O'Connell was dean of the Pittsburgh College of Pharmacy when he co-authored this manual with lawyer William Pettit. A native of Pittsburgh, O'Connell received a Ph.G. degree (1912), an A.B. (1916) and a Pharm.D. (1929) from the University of Pittsburgh, and a Pharm.M. from the Philadelphia College of Pharmacy and Science in 1932. After six years as a merchandise broker and manufacturer's agent (1916–1922), he turned to teaching at the University of Pittsburgh, holding positions from instructor to professor of chemistry, and as dean of the School of Pharmacy for fourteen years (1932–1946). He was a member of the Committee of Revision of the *United States Pharmacopoeia* (1940–50) and of several professional, scientific, and honorary societies.

Other Books: Proceedings, Surveys, Yearbooks, Studies

C46 Minutes of the convention of pharmaceutists and druggists held in the city of New York, October 15, 1851. Philadelphia: Merrihew & Son, Printers, 1865. 1 *l*, 4–11 p. 14.5×21.5 cm. Bound together with: "Proceedings of the National Pharmaceutical Convention held in Philadelphia, October 6th, 1852." Philadelphia: Merrihew & Son, Printers, (second unaltered edition) 1865. 2 *l*, 6–32 p.; "Proceedings of the American Pharmaceutical Association at the annual meeting,

held in Boston, August 24th, 25th and 26th, 1853." Philadelphia: Merrihew & Thompson, Printers, 1853. 1 *l*, 4–48 p.;
"Proceedings of the American Pharmaceutical Association at
the third annual meeting, held in Cincinnati, July 25th and
26th, 1854." Philadelphia, Merrihew & Thompson Printers,
1854. 1 *l*, 4–40 p.; "Proceedings of the American Pharmaceutical Association at the fourth annual meeting, held in New
York, September 11th, 12th and 13th, 1855." Philadelphia:
Merrihew & Son, Printers (second unaltered edition), 1865. 1
l, 4-40 p. (WU) **AIHP 36**

The *Proceedings of the American Pharmaceutical Association*
is an important class of publications in the American pharmaco-
historical literature. The volume presented here includes the minutes of the 1851 meeting preceding the foundation of the Association, the *Proceedings* of the National Pharmaceutical Convention
held the following year, during which the Association was established, and separate proceedings of its next three annual meetings
(Boston, 1853; Cincinnati, 1854; and New York, 1855). A significant
historical resource for the early stages of the professionalization of
American pharmacy, *Minutes of the Convention of Pharmaceutists*
offers a realistic view of the major concerns of pharmacy leaders,
and of their aspirations and plans to raise the level of pharmacy
practice. It is rich in detail and contains many reports and other
documents, besides giving valuable information on the early history
of the first national association of American pharmacists.

From the "importation of adulterated drugs, chemicals and
medicinal preparations" and the lack of drug standards for use by
the drug inspectors, the agenda of the meetings expanded to include
other problems. This volume contains the Constitution, Code of
Ethics, lists of members and officers of the Association, and reports,
discussions, and resolutions pertaining to many issues directly related to the improvement of pharmacy practice. It touches on matters such as standards for the use of drug inspectors, and their qualifications, home drug adulteration, local associations, schools of
pharmacy, selection and attention given to apprentices, extent of
the required preliminary education, number of apothecaries and
druggists in the different states, status of the separation of dispensing
and prescribing and of state pharmacy laws, quality of the pharmaceutical literature, and the use of the *Pharmacopoeia*.

The *Proceedings* of the annual meetings of the American Pharmaceutical Association appeared as separate volumes until 1911
(except for 1861 when no meeting occurred). Then proceedings were
published at first in three consecutive numbers of the *Journal* of
the Association, and later in one number until 1945 when printed
proceedings were discontinued (except for news reports). A useful

historical reference tool is the *General Index to Volumes One to Fifty of the Proceedings of the American Pharmaceutical Association From 1852 to 1902 Inclusive.*

From 1912 to 1934 some Association data and the Report on the Progress of Pharmacy, which used to be a part of the *Proceedings*, were published in a separate annual volume titled *Yearbook of the American Pharmaceutical Association* (see C49).

C47 OLDBERG, Oscar, 1846–1913

A course of home study for pharmacists. First lessons in the study of pharmacy. Chicago: The Apothecaries' Company, [c. 1891]. 3 *l*, v–xiv, 1 *l*, 523 p. 15×22 cm. (WU) **AIHP 44**

Home-study books were one way of preparing for state board examinations when, after the 1870s, pharmacy laws began requiring that prospective pharmacists demonstrate a certain level of knowledge, but without specifying how such knowledge should be acquired. Here is the best known example of this type of book. Its purpose was to aid those in pharmacy practice who did not have a college of pharmacy education, and to prepare others for a college course or for passing the state examinations. The author states that although "the best way to acquire a pharmaceutical education is to attend a good college of pharmacy. . ., home study is of the highest importance to those who are prevented by circumstances from entering college." This book offered preparatory home reading in physics, chemistry, materia medica, and pharmacy, paralleling courses instituted by the Northwestern University College of Pharmacy at the time the book was published. The author of the book was the dean of the College.

Subtitled "First Lessons in the Study of Pharmacy," this book gives a sense of the basic pharmaceutical knowledge expected of licensure applicants to state boards at the end of the nineteenth century. The book is divided into four parts and contains 150 illustrations. About two-thirds of the book is devoted to Elements of Pharmaceutical Physics (Part I) and Elements of Chemistry (Part II), the rest to Materia Medica (Part III) and Pharmacy (Part IV). Each part is subdivided into chapters. Some examples of the subject matter are: definitions of terms, plant constituents, vegetable crude drugs (under a morphological classification), animal drugs, therapeutic classification of medicines, doses of nearly 1,000 articles, pharmacy apparatus and processes, general review of pharmaceutical preparations and preparations by classes (powders, pills, syrups, abstracts, suppositories, and many others), pharmaceutical nomenclature, and weights and measures.

One other edition was published (1896, reprinted in 1898). This volume replaced the author's earlier *Outline of a Course in Practical Pharmacy*, also designed for home-study.

Born in Sweden, Oscar Oldberg, received his early education there and came to the United States when he was eighteen years old. Eventually he became engaged in educational and literary activities, notably as a member of the Committee of Revision of the United States *Pharmacopoeia* (1880), and professor of pharmacy, director of pharmaceutical laboratories and dean of the Northwestern University College of Pharmacy (1886–1911). His other publications include *A Companion to the United States Pharmacopoeia* (with Otto A. Wall, 1884), *Fifteen Hundred Examples of Prescriptions and Formulas* (1892), and *Inorganic Chemistry, General, Medical and Pharmaceutical* (1900).

C48 The pharmaceutical syllabus. First edition recommended by the National Committee representing the boards and schools of pharmacy of the United States for the first syllabus period of August 1, 1910 to July 31, 1915. n.p.: J. B. Lyon Co., Printers, 1910. 1 *l*, 4–146 p. 14.5×21.5 cm. (WU) **AIHP 53**

This publication marks the emergence of the curricular literature of American pharmacy. For use by the schools of pharmacy and the boards of pharmacy, it introduced "a *minimum course* of study and a syllabus for the guidance of pharmacy schools in their preparation of students for admission to the boards' licensing examinations." A valuable historical source, this work paved the way for: (1) a definition of education for pharmacists and of sound licensing examinations; (2) a feasible degree of uniformity in the minimum requirements of the boards and in the minimum instruction of the schools; and (3) a closer connection between the boards and the schools in meeting their respective goals.

Prepared from subjects found in state board examinations and in the curriculum of pharmacy schools, the *Pharmaceutical Syllabus* proposed a two-year course of 1,000 hours, divided into three branches: materia medica (nine subjects, 300 hours) including physiology, botany, pharmacognosy, pharmaco- and therapy-dynamics; chemistry (nine subjects, 400 hours) comprised by elementary physics, elementary chemistry, qualitative chemistry, manufacturing chemistry, drug assaying, and others; and pharmacy (eight subjects, 300 hours) including pharmaceutical arithmetic, pharmaceutical Latin, theory of pharmacy, practice of pharmacy, commercial pharmacy, manufacturing pharmacy, dispensing pharmacy, and pharmaceutical jurisprudence. Those interested in education found here subject outlines, laboratory experiments, and definitions of pharmaceutical terms. The first year was envisioned to prepare students for examination as licensed druggists or licensed assistants, and the second year for examination as licensed pharmacists.

This manual was prepared by the National Syllabus Committee representing the nation's boards and schools of pharmacy and the American Pharmaceutical Association. The twenty-one-member committee was organized in September 1906 under leadership by the New York board, which sought to identify an adequate pharmacy standard to comply with a 1905 New York law, the first to require a college diploma for pharmacy licensure. The completed *Pharmaceutical Syllabus* was approved by the New York State Board of Pharmacy in January 1910 and distributed nationally to the members of all boards of pharmacy and to administrators of the schools of pharmacy. It was recommended for the First Syllabus Period, August 1, 1910 to July 31, 1915.

Other editions appeared in 1913, 1922, and 1932 (which introduced the four-year program). In 1945 a tentative mimeographed version was issued just before dissolution of the Committee.

C49 Year book of the American Pharmaceutical Association 1912. Scio, OH: The American Pharmaceutical Association, 1914. 1 *l*, v–xl, 621 p. 14.5×22 cm. (WU) **AIHP 83**

Concurrent with discontinuation of the *Proceedings* of the annual meetings of the American Pharmaceutical Association (see C46), was the publication of the *Year Book*, compiling the Report on the Progress of Pharmacy and some Association data in one volume. The first issue, presented here, corresponds to volume sixty of the former *Proceedings* and contains the 1912 Report, and the Constitution, By-Laws, and membership roster of the Association. At the time it was envisioned that the Report "as a separate and distinct annual volume" would "prove of inestimable value to the average practicing pharmacist as a work of daily reference." Today it is a valuable historical resource.

Consisting of abstracts of original papers published in German and American journals, the Report is in effect a literature survey covering in this issue nearly 400 topics on pharmacy, materia medica, and inorganic and organic chemistry. The abstracts listed under pharmacy deal with apparatus and manipulations, preparations, and new remedies and trade name preparations; under materia medica, with vegetable and animal drug products; under inorganic chemistry, with non-metallic elements and metals; and under organic chemistry, it covers hydrocarbons (including volatile oils), alcohol and derivatives, carbohydrates, glucosides, coloring matters, and so on.

For more than thirty years the leading force behind the Report had been the versatile German-born American pharmacist, research worker, and teacher, C. Lewis Diehl (1840–1917), who died about three years after the Report was first included in the *Year Book*. Other younger collaborators in this issue included well-known pharmacists Henry V. Arny, Otto Raubenheimer, and Martin I. Wilbert.

C50 CHARTERS, W[erret] W[allace] et al., 1875–1952

Basic material for a pharmaceutical curriculum. New York and London: McGraw-Hill Book Co., Inc., 1927. xiii, 366 p. 14×22 cm. (WU) **AIHP 07**

This book was the report of the first pharmaceutical survey in the United States based on the principle of task analysis of the practice of pharmacy. With more effective pharmaceutical education as its objective, *Basic Material for a Pharmaceutical Curriculum* was published when *The Pharmaceutical Syllabus* (see C48) was in its third edition. However, in the work presented here an attempt was made for the first time to outline the education and training of community pharmacists in terms of duties performed by them. Paving the way for a four-year minimum curriculum, it had a positive effect on the profession of pharmacy and a meaningful influence on teaching.

The outcome of a unified national effort by the American Association of Colleges of Pharmacy, the National Association of Retail Druggists, and the National Association of Boards of Pharmacy, the report was founded on twenty-six studies, which considered the community pharmacist's performance from at least eleven perspectives (e.g., as a professional, as a business person, as a compounder of prescriptions, as a manufacturer, as a defender of public health), and sought to determine what the pharmacist's knowledge should have been in over thirty subjects (e.g., jurisprudence, ethics, compounding and dispensing, mathematics, operative pharmacy, bio-assaying, pharmacology and physiology, and merchandise information). These studies, which included an assessment of standard equipment for practice, a survey of retail pharmacies, and an ingredients survey, put forward a "minimum essential content" for a curriculum, without organizing it into courses.

The text is in three sections. Section I introduces the report. Section II consists of the content of the curriculum, divided into four branches: I Pharmacy, including twelve subjects, such as compounding and dispensing, English, jurisprudence, operative pharmacy, preservation, professional morale, and techniques involved in compounding, dispensing and operative pharmacy; II Materia Medica, eleven topics (e.g., bacteriology and immunology, biological assaying, pharmacognosy, pharmacology, and public health); III Chemistry, i.e., chemistry and physics; and IV Commercial pharmacy, including merchandise information, salesmanship, and three lists—ingredients in prescriptions, standard equipment, and inventories. Section III discusses the techniques of curriculum construction.

This publication was superseded in the late 1940s by *The General Report of the Pharmaceutical Survey 1946–1949*, a study of lasting influence underwritten by the American Foundation of Pharmaceutical Education and conducted by the American Council on Education.

Basic Material for a Pharmaceutical Curriculum was prepared under the direction of Werret Wallace Charters, a well-known professor and researcher in education, at the time associated with the University of Pittsburgh. Professors A. Bertram Lemon and Leon M. Monell of the University of Buffalo were associate directors in the project. Robert P. Fischelis, then Secretary and Chemist of the Board of Pharmacy of the State of New Jersey, edited the manuscript, prepared the index, and saw the material through publication. The list of contributors includes the best-known names in American pharmacy, for example, H. C. Christensen, R. A. Lyman, H. H. Rusby, J. Leon Lascoff, James H. Beal, E. Fullerton Cook, C. H. LaWall, H. V. Arny, P. S. Pittenger, Wilbur L. Scoville, E. N. Gathercoal, Torald Sollman, and Edward Kremers. Several manufacturing laboratories, at least thirty-four schools and colleges of pharmacy, and over a thousand practicing pharmacists also contributed to the findings.

C51 National Conference on Pharmaceutical Research, 1928/ 29–1932/33. No place or date of publication. 372 p. Each year paginated separately. 13.5×20.5 cm. (WU) **AIHP 40**

This book is a unique record of research in progress in American pharmacy during a five-year period in the late 1920s and early 1930s. It contains the fifth through ninth annual census of the National Conference on Pharmaceutical Research. The first four (1924/ 25 to 1927/28) had appeared consecutively in volumes fourteen to seventeen of the *Journal of the American Pharmaceutical Association.*

Compiled through questionnaires sent to numerous institutions, such as schools and colleges of pharmacy, drug manufacturers, and government agencies, the book lists pharmaceutical research in at least eleven categories. Included are bacteriology, business, pharmacology and bio-assays, history, and pharmaceutical physics, as well as dispensing pharmacy, standardization of U.S.P. and N.F. galenicals, manufacture of medicinal chemicals, sources and identification of botanic drugs, and chemistry of drug plants. The latter topics constitute the greater part of the work.

After a roster of conference and committee members, there is a list of over 400 research workers with their affiliations, locations (towns), and subjects under investigation, for each of the five years. The researchers come from all parts of the nation. About two-thirds were pharmacy teachers and their students, and manufacturing pharmacists; these were followed in number by chemists, botanists, and pharmacologists, and by some practicing pharmacists and others. Random examples of the types of subjects covered would be chemistry of the seeds of *Lansium domesticum*, identification of shrimp oil, U.S.P. methods of analysis, preservation of tincture of aconite, alkaloidal indicators, and the quality of drugs and pharmaceuticals.

From 1933–34 the proceedings issues of the Conference were supplanted by yearly reports under the title *Annual Survey of Research in Pharmacy and Proceedings of the National Conference on Pharmaceutical Research*. Published until 1940, they presented the growth of pharmaceutical research in a narrative style, documented with many references.

The National Conference on Pharmaceutical Research was brought into being in 1922 by the American Association of Colleges of Pharmacy, the American Drug Manufacturers Association, and the American Pharmaceutical Association, as founding members. One of its functions was to "aid in coordinating the research activities of its members and to encourage pharmaceutical research in its broadest sense." In the 1930s its sixteen members included additional organizations such as the Bureau of Chemistry of the U.S. Department of Agriculture, the National Association of Boards of Pharmacy, the U.S.P. and N.F. revision committees, the Plant Science Seminar, and the Hygienic Laboratory of the U.S. Public Health Service.

C52 ROREM, C[larence] Rufus, b. 1894 and FISCHELIS, Robert P., 1891–1981

The costs of medicines. The manufacture and distribution of drugs and medicines in the United States and the services of pharmacy in medical care. Publication No. 14 of the Committee on the Costs of Medical Care. Chicago: University of Chicago Press, [c. 1932]. xi, 250 p., 3 *l*. 15×21 cm. (WU) **AIHP 65**

This book is the report of a comprehensive fact-finding survey made under the auspices of the Committee on the Costs of Medical Care, designed to record and interpret the professional and commercial interests of the manufacture and distribution of medicines in the United States. Meanwhile it has become a valuable historical source on the economic aspects of "pharmacal" care in the late 1920s and early 1930s.

The book is divided into three parts, with thirteen chapters and six appendices. Part I, "Pharmacy and Medical Care" (Chapters I–III), deals with such topics as the definition and early history and development of pharmacy, average family expenditures for medicines, number and distribution of registered pharmacists, incomes and professional opportunities of pharmacists, and costs of pharmaceutical education. Part II, "Pharmacy and the Drug Industry" (Chapters IV–X), covers areas such as the number of pharmacies and gross sales, distribution of pharmacies, the prescription practice, financial organization and operation of the pharmacy, financial organization and operation of the pharmacy, other retail dispensers of medicines, types of drug manufacturers, and "big business" in the manufacture of medicines. Part III, "Pharmacy and the Public" (Chapters XI–XIII), includes legislative control of drugs and medicines, state licensure and governmental regulation of pharmacists and pharmacies, professional control of drugs and medicines, the physician's use of pharmacy, economic friction between physicians and pharmacists, and so on. Chapter XIII contains a summary, conclusion, and the authors' recommendations. Statistical data are presented mostly by means of sixteen tables. One appendix consists of the Code of Ethics of the American Pharmaceutical Association (1922). The others contain data on tuition, enrollment and degree requirements of the schools of pharmacy as of 1930; provisions of the pharmacy laws for the sale of proprietary and patent medicines, and of non-proprietary medicines; location of drug stores; and minimum state requirements for the practice of pharmacy.

The Committee on the Costs of Medical Care was organized in 1927 in Washington, D.C., at a conference called by ten physicians, three economists, and three non-medical persons working in the public health field. Its purpose was "to study the economic aspects of the prevention and care of sickness, including the adequacy, availability, and compensation of the persons and agencies concerned." The Committee received significant assistance from many agencies (e.g., American Medical Association, National Bureau of Economic Research, U.S. Public Health Service) and economic support from institutions like the Carnegie and Rockefeller foundations. The authors were members of the research staff engaged by the Committee.

A native of Iowa, Clarence Rufus Rorem was an economist and certified public accountant with A.M. and Ph.D. degrees from the University of Chicago. Active for many years in the study of medical care problems, and particularly interested in pre-payment of health services, he was the author of about twenty books and brochures and over 100 articles. Rorem received several awards from hospital-related organizations.

Born in Philadelphia, Robert Philip Fischelis received Ph.G., Ph.C., B.Sc., and Pharm.D. degrees from the Medico-Chirurgical College of Philadelphia, and became one of the most influential pharmacists of the present century. Holding various positions of leadership during his long career, he was especially interested in pharmaceutical education, journalism, and regulation, and in pharmacy affairs nationally. His appointments included serving as Secretary and Chief Chemist of the New Jersey Board of Pharmacy for eighteen years (1926–1944), a position held while he co-authored the present book, as Secretary and General Manager of the American Pharmaceutical Association for fourteen years (1945–1959), and as Dean of the College of Pharmacy of Ohio Northern University (1963–1965). He also served in such organizations as the American Association of Colleges of Pharmacy, the American Council on Pharmaceutical Education, the National Research Council, the *United States Pharmacopoeia*, and the National Association of Boards of Pharmacy.

For his numerous and diverse contributions to pharmacy, he received the Remington Medal, several honorary degrees, and other recognitions.

C53 GATHERCOAL, E[dmund] N[orris], 1874–1954

> The prescription ingredient survey. Consisting of: The Ebert survey 1885; Hallberg survey 1895; Hallberg-Snow survey 1907; Charters survey 1926; Cook survey 1930; Gathercoal survey 1930; U.S.P.-N.F. survey 1931–32. n.p.: The American Pharmaceutical Association, 1933. 172 p. 17×25 cm. (WU) **AIHP 19**

This book puts together the results of seven surveys showing the trends in the use and character of prescription drugs over a period of nearly five decades from the early 1880s to the early 1930s. Other contemporary surveys, such as the National Drug Store Survey, 1930–1931,* and one of the studies of the Committee on the Costs of Medical Care (see C52), presented interesting data on drugs and medicines, but dealt mostly with their costs, distribution and

---

*A series of eight studies of drug store operations made by the U.S. Department of Commerce and published as bulletins of the Bureau of Foreign and Domestic Commerce between 1932 and 1934. Included are monographs on *Drug Store Arrangement, Wholesale Druggists' Operations, Merchandising in City Drug Stores, Merchandising in Country Drug Stores, Merchandising Requirements of the Drug Store Package, Prescription Department Sales Analysis in Selected Drug Stores, Costs, Sales, and Profits in the Retail Drug Store,* and *Causes of Failure among Drug Stores.*

extent of use, not with their nature or type. The surveys considered here offer a remarkably concrete picture of prescription practice as it evolved over nearly a half century, and were useful in the revision of the *Pharmacopoeia* and of the *National Formulary*. They are: The Ebert Survey of 1885, The Hallberg Survey of 1895, The Hallberg-Snow Survey of 1907, The Charters Survey of 1926, The Cook Survey of 1930, The Gathercoal Survey of 1930, and The U.S.P.-N.F. Survey of 1931–1932.

The results of these studies (originally prepared in different formats, with variations in definitions and scope, and some unpublished) have been combined in the present volume so that they can be easily compared. The book is arranged in five parts. Part I contains a brief description and summary of each survey. Part II discusses some unique features of the seven surveys, for example, the number of components in the prescriptions, classification of the drugs and medicines, items of highest occurrence, and comparison of official and non-official products. Part III explains the principles guiding the USP-NF Survey. Part IV, the major part of the book, consists of an alphabetical tabulation of the thousands of ingredients mentioned in the seven surveys, showing the incidence of each ingredient per 10,000 prescriptions in each survey. Part V is a cross reference to the ingredients listed in the seven surveys.

Edmund Norris Gathercoal was born in Illinois. Having received a Ph.G. degree from the Chicago College of Pharmacy in 1895, he practiced retail pharmacy for twelve years. Gathercoal was associated with the Chicago College of Pharmacy for nearly five decades, beginning in 1907 as instructor in botany and pharmacognosy, then as professor (1924), and finally as professor emeritus. In 1934 he received a Pharm.M. degree from the Philadelphia College of Pharmacy. His professional commitments included membership in the Committee on Revision of the U.S.P. for two decades (1920–1940), chairmanship of the National Conference on Pharmaceutical Research (see C51), and, at the time he compiled the present book, chairmanship of the National Formulary Revision Committee, and presidency of the American Pharmaceutical Association in 1938. Contributing over thirty publications to the pharmaceutical literature, he was joint editor of the third edition (1928) of Kraemer's *Scientific and Applied Pharmacognosy* (see C26) and co-author of a textbook based on the latter, *Pharmacognosy*, published in 1936. In recognition of his research contributions, he was awarded the Ebert Prize in 1914 and held membership in several honorary societies.

C54 Year book of the American Pharmaceutical Association 1934. Washington, D.C.: American Pharmaceutical Association, 1936. 1 *l*, xxxix, 1 *l*, 3–468 p. 14.5×22 cm. (WU) **AIHP**
84

This is the final volume of a special category of pharmaceutical literature that for over twenty years reported what was going on in American pharmacy, and remains today a significant historical source. It contains the 1934 (Seventy-Seventh) Report on the Progress of Pharmacy, as well as the Constitution, By-Laws, and other Association data.

Reduced to about three-fourths of the size of the first volume (see C49), the 1934 Report reflects the changes occuring in the practice of pharmacy by the fourth decade of the century. Although abstracts on only about forty topics (in contrast to nearly 400 in the first report) appear under the general categories of pharmacy, materia medica, and chemistry, new subjects are introduced under these headings. For example, under pharmacy: pharmaceutical history, education, and legislation; pharmacopoeias and formularies; dispensing, hospital and commercial pharmacy, and technical recipes. Under materia medica: pharmacognosy, medicinal plant culture; organotherapeutic agents, enzymes, serums, and vaccines; new remedies—synthetic, chemotherapeutic, antiseptics, and disinfectants; pharmacology, toxicology, and therapeutics, including physiological standardization. Under chemistry: analytical chemistry, which comprises over one-half of the section.

After the demise of the *Year Book* a modified version of the Report titled "Pharmaceutical Abstracts" appeared monthly in the *Journal* of the Association through 1939, and in the *Scientific Edition* of the *Journal* until 1948. Association data and the roster, which were part of the *Year Book*, subsequently were also published in the *Journal*.

D. TRADE CATALOGS*

Brief notations on thirteen selected trade catalogs are presented here, portraying the wares sold by pharmaceutical manufacturers, wholesalers, and retailers in the United States from the late colonial period to the fourth decade of the twentieth century.

As early as the founding of the Republic, trade catalogs began emerging as significant advertising and marketing instruments of the trades, specialized crafts, and professions, and today they are useful in tracing economic, technological, and social aspects of these occupations. Pharmaceutical trade catalogs feature shop and laboratory furniture, apparatus, glassware, drugstore sundries, crude drugs, galenicals, patent medicines, prescription specialties, and chemicals. Collectors and historical researchers find these catalogs

*Part of the information in this section was taken from Griffenhagen, G. B. and L. B. Romaine, "Early U.S. Pharmaceutical Catalogues," *Am. J. Pharm.* 131 (1959):14–33.

valuable in identifying the stock and fittings of the pharmacy establishment of the past, for determining the dates of origin, periods of use, the manufacturers and distributors, and for comparative studies of the terminology, types, and variety of drugs in demand, and the cost of the stock in drugstores.

Before the American Revolution merchants generally advertised their commodities in newspapers or through broadsides intended primarily to promote sales of a single product. Pharmacy broadsides dealt mostly with individual patent medicines, although a broadside issued about 1725 advertised a variety of medicines, and has been described as the first individual publication by an American pharmacist in British America—"A Catalogue of Medicines Sold by Mr. Robert Talbot of Burlington." In the few actual trade catalogs issued during this period, articles were listed without printed prices. Two pharmaceutical examples are known: *A Catalogue of Druggs and of chymical and Galenical Medicines; Sold by John Tweedy at his Shop in Newport, Rhode Island. And for him in New-York at the Sign of the Unicorn and Mortar*, which is among the first catalogs of any type issued in this country. It is a twenty-eight-page alphabetical list by Latin names of about 580 chemicals and galenicals, apparently issued between 1757 and 1760, which copied the style and format of earlier English catalogs. The other known colonial catalog of this kind is the Day, *Catalogue of Drugs* (1771) (see D1).

The first pharmaceutical trade catalogs of the Republic were issued by wholesale druggists. Until the late 1820s the articles were listed without printed prices, like their colonial predecessors. Up to the 1830s the catalogs generally had less than forty pages, but by the 1850s they generally had over 100 pages. Until the 1850s the catalogs seldom carried illustrations, but from the 1870s they were richly illustrated, and became sizeable and well-bound volumes that mirrored the realities of the pharmaceutical shop or laboratory.

D1 John Day and Co.
Catalogue of drugs, chymical and galenical preparations, shop furniture, patent medicines, and surgeon instruments . . . Philadelphia: John Dunlap, Printer, 1771. 29 p. (Evans 12024) (PPAmP)

Of two known pharmaceutical trade catalogs of the Colonial period, this one provides a picture of the stock and fittings of the American pharmacy establishment before the Revolution. It consists almost entirely (about twenty-three pages) of a list of nearly 790 galenicals and chemicals by their Latin names (items such as ipecac, cantharides, and Peruvian bark; calomel and tartar emetic; viper's fat and crab claws; and English patent medicines such as the widely sold Anderson's Pills and Bateman's Pectoral Drops). Also included are some shop furniture and surgical instruments, drug sundries like tooth brushes and tooth powder, nipple shells, urinals, and enema pipes (glysters), and a variety of colognes. The articles were listed without printed prices, but blank columns permitted prices and quantities to be inserted.

D2 Smith and Bartlett (firm)
Catalogue of drugs and medicines, instruments and utensils, dye-stuffs, groceries and painters' colours, imported, prepared, and sold by Smith & Bartlett at their druggists stores and apothecaries shop, Boston. Boston: Manning & Loring, Printers, 1795. 22 p. 11×17.5 cm. (Evans 29537) (MBCP) **AIHP 70**

This catalog of the early national period was selected to illustrate the stock advertised by an importer-manufacturer-wholesaler-dispenser of drugs and medicines at the end of the eighteenth century. The Smith and Bartlett *Catalogue of Drugs and Medicines* lists about 270 drugs and preparations in alphabetical order by Latin names, about thirty English patent medicines (such as Anderson's Pills, Bateman's Pectoral Drops, and Godfrey's Cordial), surgeon's instruments, and miscellaneous sundries (such as tooth brushes, nutgalls, scales and weights, and pill boxes). Like the Colonial catalogs, printed prices are not included.

The stock does not differ greatly from John Day's catalog of two decades earlier (see D1), but it adds such items as utensils, dye-stuffs, groceries, and painter's colors that were ordinarily imported, prepared, and sold through druggists' stores and apothecary shops at the time, and into the nineteenth century.

D3 T[homas] W. Dyott (firm)
Approved patent and family medicines, which are celebrated for the cure of most diseases to which the human body is liable . . . for sale in Philadelphia only at the proprietors wholesale and retail drug and family medicine warehouse . . . Philadelphia, 1814. 28 p. 13.5×21.5 cm. (Evans 31384) (WU) **AIHP 14**

This publication exemplifies trade catalogs put out by the large drug "warehouses" during the first half of the nineteenth century, which sold such articles as patent medicines, drugs, chemicals, sundries, and nostrums both at wholesale and retail. Thomas W. Dyott, one of the first merchandisers to develop a national market for his products, had one of the more successful drug merchandising and manufacturing enterprises of the early nineteenth century, selling his own brands as well as English and other American brands of patent medicines.

The catalog lists thirteen of Dyott's medicines "for the cure of most diseases to which the human body is liable," bearing the name of a Dr. Robertson, allegedly a famous Edinburgh physician, and Dyott's grandfather. Also included, without printed prices, are about 240 drugs and close to fifty patent medicines, as well as chemicals, dye-stuffs, paints, sundries, and glass articles such as tincture bottles, funnels, and "sucking" bottles.

D4 The druggist's manual. Being a price current of drugs, medicines, paints, dye-stuffs, glass, patent medicines, etc., with Latin and English synonyms, a German, French, and Spanish catalogue of drugs, etc. Compiled by direction of the Philadelphia College of Pharmacy. Philadelphia: Solomon W. Conrad, Printer, 1826. xvii, 119 p. 13.5×22 cm. (WU) **AIHP 12**

This is the first "price current" of its kind representing an endeavor of the Philadelphia College of Pharmacy as a local association to disseminate current scientific and professional information useful to practitioners of pharmacy.

A list of about 850 drugs, arranged alphabetically by Latin names, constitutes the main section of the book. Next are a list of some 100 patent medicines, and lists of glassware, surgeon's instruments, paints and dye-stuffs, and miscellaneous articles, all with blank columns for the prices to be written in. Other information includes English and Latin names and synonyms; French, Spanish, and German names of some drugs; and twenty-one tables selected "to make scientific accuracy the habit and characteristic of the Trade."

D5 T. Morris Perot and Co.
Prices current for druggists only. Drugs, medicines, chemicals, etc. Philadelphia: no publ., [c. 1857 or c. 1858] 52 p. 13×21 cm. (WU) **AIHP 51**

One of the early illustrated American pharmaceutical trade catalogs, this one emphasizes the representation of specific brands and products of importers and wholesale dealers acting as exclusive agents for specified manufacturers. It represents the pharmaceutical trade catalogs that began appearing in the 1850s. In addition to the usual wares—such as paints, oils, miscellaneous articles and instruments, and druggists' glasswares—this catalog offered solid and fluid extracts and other preparations manufactured by a specific company (Tilden & Co., New Lebanon, NY). It also featured soda, mineral water and syrup apparatus of a specific manufacturer (the Nichol's Mineral Water Fountain).

D6 McKesson & Robbins (firm)
Prices current of drugs and druggists' articles, chemical and pharmaceutical preparations, proprietary medicines and perfumery, sponges, corks, dyes, paints, etc. New York: Thitchener and Glastaeter, Printers, 1872. 3 *l*, 8–128 p. 14.5×21 cm. (WU) **AIHP 34**

This illustrated catalog exemplifies the type and variety of the merchandise stocked by large American wholesale drug establishments of the 1870s. The first twenty-seven pages form the price book, and were printed so that price changes could be inserted. They include the medicinal and technical drugs commonly requested (in alphabetical sequence), classified into acids, barks, extracts, flowers, gums, leaves, oils, roots, and seeds. Listed separately are such items as rare drugs, chemicals, and pharmaceutical preparations; pressed herbs, roots, and barks; concentrated medicines; gelatin-coated and sugar-coated pills; French and English proprietary articles; concentrated essences; pure fruit juices; and the McKesson & Robbins brands of fluid extracts, elixirs, specialties, and other products. Also included are surgical appliances; druggists' sundries such as corks, glassware, paper, scales and twines; brushes, combs, and perfumery; paints and colors; window glass; smokers' articles; guns and sporting materials; and metal show cases. The inclusion of tests to determine the adulteration of essential oils with turpentine, fixed oils, alcohol or other essential oils is unique for this kind of publication.

D7 Whitall, Tatum and Co.
Glass manufacture. Druggists' sundries. Philadelphia and New York: no publ., 1880. 72 p. 15.5×23 cm. (WU) **AIHP 78**

Typical of the richly illustrated American catalogs of the 1880s, this issue has been selected to portray mainly the products of a leading manufacturer of druggists', chemists', and perfumers' glassware. Its nearly 200 different categories of wares include stoppers; flint, blue, and green glassware; pomade containers and glass bottles; homeopathic vials; show bottles and globes; fruit jars; and chemical ware, as well as druggists' sundries, shop and prescription-desk furniture, and scales. The series of this catalog, continuing at least to 1899, is one of the best references to American glass.

D8 James W. Tufts (firm)
Arctic soda water apparatus. Boston, [c. 1888]. 2 *l*, 5–220 p. 18.5×24 cm. (WU) **AIHP 74**

Originating in Europe in the late eighteenth and early nineteenth centuries, soda water and carbonated fruit beverages were soon popularized in the United States, and counter dispensing of effervescent fruit drinks by the glass became a common practice in drug stores. Ornate fountains appeared in the 1860s, and by the 1880s the soda fountain was an American institution.

The illustrated catalog presented here is actually a handbook intended for dispensers, bottlers, and manufacturers of carbonated beverages. Besides prices for the apparatus and their parts, it gives directions for setting up and operating them, as well as recipes for syrups and drinks, and miscellaneous receipts, such as cement for white marble, and a solution for cleaning silverware.

D9 Henry Heil Chemical Company
Illustrated catalogue and price-list of chemical and physical apparatus and instruments for laboratories, chemists, iron and steel works, smelters, . . . schools, colleges, universities, etc. St. Louis: no publ., [c. 1891]. 2 *l*, 10–447 p. 16×24.5 cm. (WU) **AIHP 22**

This is one of the early large catalogs featuring general laboratory apparatus and instruments for chemists, iron and steel works, smelters, assayers, mines, sugar refineries, schools, colleges, universities, and so on. Although not precisely a pharmaceutical trade catalog, it offered for sale many appliances and utensils used in chemical and pharmacy laboratories of the late nineteenth century. Amply illustrated, it includes such items as polarizers and polarizing tubes, hydraulic presses, flasks, forceps, crucibles, balances, air pumps, and apparatus for the analysis of gases.

D10 Peter Van Schaack and Sons
Annual price current. Drugs, chemicals, medicines. Chicago: J. M. W. Jones Stationery and Printing Co., Printers, 1899. 5 *l*, 7-1116 p. 11.5x18 cm. (WU) **AIHP 75**

This catalog shows the turn-of-the-century stock and the merchandising policies of an important import-export-wholesale establishment, founded in the early 1840s away from the eastern seaports. Its diversified offerings include pharmaceutical preparations, with descriptions and uses; chemical products; acids and mineral waters; paints, oils and varnishes; toilet articles; proprietary medicines; and soda fountain supplies. Adding to its usefulness as a historical source are many pictures and drawings of prescription cases, glass labels, glassware in general, scales, thermometers, surgical instruments, and so on.

D11 M. Winter Lumber Company
Winter's Catalogue - No. 87. Commercial furniture; drug, jewelry and cigar store fixtures. Sheboygan, WI: no publ., 1910. 1 *l*, B–Q, x, xx, 2 *l*, 320–629 p. 22.5×30 cm. (WU) **AIHP 81**

Over half of this unique catalog is devoted to pharmacy furniture, highlighting drug store fixtures such as prescription-case partitions and counters, as well as shelving for patent medicines, tinctures, and sundries. It also advertises soda fountains, and fountain counters. Twelve pages of floor plans and sixty full-page pictures of pharmacy interiors fitted by the manufacturer portray some of the finest midwestern establishments of the early twentieth century.

D12 Wm. S. Merrell Company
Complete descriptive catalog of pharmaceutical preparations and ethical specialties. Cincinnati, [c. 1918]. 1 *l*, 5–200 p. 12×19.5 cm. (WU) **AIHP 35**

Available only to a "physician or druggist," this catalog was singled out to illustrate the marketing of specialties and preparations not intended for sale directly to the general public, by one of the oldest pharmaceutical manufacturing establishments in the United States.

With only a few illustrations, it lists over 900 specialties and preparations, alphabetically arranged, including narcotics and classified pharmaceuticals, such as alkaloids, resinoids, ampoules and elixirs. Numbered in sequence, the description, composition and use of each item is given. Prices appear by the number of each item in separate "Prices Current" issued periodically.

D13 S. B. Penick & Company
Price list and manual of botanical crude drugs from
the four corners of the earth. New York and Chicago,
August 1, 1938. 48 p. 11×19.5 cm. (WU) **AIHP 50**

This catalog represents the spectrum of crude drugs being offered in the late 1930s by the best known botanical house in the
United States. It lists alphabetically nearly 900 foreign and domestic
crude drugs, mostly botanical, but including such minerals as ca-
lamine and zinc oxide. The information under each item indicates
whether it had been recognized by the U.S.P. or N.F., the Latin and
common names, the uses and plant parts used, how supplied and
prices.

S. B. Penick's nineteenth-century analog was the Shakers' medicinal herbs enterprise that marked the beginning of the U. S.
botanical industry. Founded about 1820, and issuing herb catalogs
by 1830, their label was a sign of reliability and quality for over a
century.

PART TWO: CHRONOLOGICAL LIST OF SOURCES BY PUBLICATION DATES

A1 CULPEPER, Nicholas, 1616–1654

Pharmacopoeia Londinensis; or, the London dispensatory further adorned by the studies and collections of the fellows now living of the said college. Boston: John Allen, Printer, **1720.** [24], 305 p., [35]. 11.5×18.5 cm. (Evans 2114) (DNLM) **AIHP 09**

D1 John Day and Co.

Catalogue of drugs, chymical and galenical preparations, shop furniture, patent medicines, and surgeon instruments . . . Philadelphia: John Dunlap, Printer, **1771.** 29 p. (Evans 12024) (PPAmP)

C12 CULLEN, William, 1710–1790

Lectures on the materia medica as delivered by William Cullen, M.D., professor of medicine in the University of Edinburgh. Now published by permission of the author, and with many corrections from the collation of different manuscripts by the editors. Philadelphia: Robert Bell, Printer, **1775.** viii, 512 p. 19×24 cm. (Evans 14000) (WU) **AIHP 08**

B1 [BROWN, William], 1748–1792

Pharmacopoeia simpliciorum et efficaciorum in usum nosocomii militaris. Philadelphia: Styner & Cist., **1778.** 4–32 p. 9.5×16 cm. (Evans 15750) (DNLM) **AIHP 06**

A2 The Edinburgh new dispensatory. Containing I The Elements of pharmaceutical chemistry. II The Materia medica. III The Pharmaceutical and medicinal compositions of the new editions of the London (1788) and Edinburgh (1783) pharmacopoeias. Philadelphia: T. Dobson, Printer, **1791.** 3 *l*, vii–xxii, 33–656 p. 12.5×20 cm. (Evans 23503) (WU) **AIHP 16**

D2 Smith and Bartlett (firm)

Catalogue of drugs and medicines, instruments and utensils, dye-stuffs, groceries and painters' colours, imported, prepared, and sold by Smith & Bartlett at their druggists stores and apothecaries shop, Boston. Boston: Manning & Loring, Printers, **1795**. 22 p. 11×17.5 cm. (Evans 29537) (MBCP) **AIHP 70**

C13 MURRAY, J[ohn], 1778–1820

Elements of materia medica and pharmacy. Two vols. in one. Philadelphia: B. and T. Kite, **1808**. vi–xii, 13–447 p. 12.5×20 cm. (Evans 15670) (WU) **AIHP 39**

B2 The pharmacopoeia of the Massachusetts Medical Society. Boston: E. & J. Larkin, **1808**. 3 *l*, v–x, 2 *l*, 3–272 p. 10×18 cm. (Evans 15554) (WU) **AIHP 56**

C14 BARTON, Benjamin Smith, 1766–1815

Collections for an essay towards a materia medica of the United States. Third edition. Philadelphia: Edward Earle and Co., **1810**. Part first: 2 *l*, v–xvi, 3–67 p. Part second: 1 *l*, iii–xv, 53 p. 12.5×21 cm. (Evans 19478) (WU) **AIHP 02**

A3 THACHER, James, 1754–1844

The American new dispensatory. Containing general principles of pharmaceutic chemistry. Pharmaceutic operations. Chemical analysis of the articles of materia medica. Materia medica including several new and valuable articles, the production of the United States. Preparations and compositions . . . . Boston: T. B. Wait & Co., **1810**. 3 *l*, 7–529 p. 13×20 cm. (Evans 21476) (WU) **AIHP 72**

C28 SMITH, Peter, 1753–1816

The Indian doctor's dispensatory, being Father Smith's advice respecting diseases and their cure; consisting of prescriptions for many complaints; and a description of medicines, simple and compound, showing their virtues and how to apply them. Designed for the benefit of his children, his friends and the public, but more especially the citizens of the western parts of the United States of America. Cincinatti: Browne and Looker, Printers, **1813**. i–iv, 108 p. 17.1×10 cm. (OCLloyd)

D3 T[homas] W. Dyott (firm)

Approved patent and family medicines, which are celebrated for the cure of most diseases to which the human body is liable . . . for sale in Philadelphia only at the proprietors wholesale and retail drug and family medicine warehouse . . . Philadelphia, **1814**. 28 p. 13.5×21.5 cm. (Evans 31384) (WU) **AIHP 14**

B3 Pharmacopoeia nosocomii Neo-Eboracensis; or the pharmacopoeia of the New York Hospital . . . an appendix containing a general posological table and a comparative view of the former and present terms in materia medica and pharmacy. New York: Collins & Co., **1816**. 2 *l*, vi–x, 1 *l*, 180, 1 p. 12×20 cm. (Evans 38453) (WU) **AIHP 57**

C15 BARTON, William P[aul] C[rillon], 1786–1856

Vegetable materia medica of the United States, or medical botany: containing a botanical, general, and medical history of medicinal plants indigenous to the United States. Illustrated by coloured engravings made after original drawings from nature, done by the author. Two vols. Philadelphia: M. Carey & Son, vol. 1 **1817**; vol. 2 **1818**. Vol. 1: 3 *l*, vi–xv, 17–273 p. 21×26.5 cm. Vol 2: 3 *l*, viii–xvi, 9–243 p. 21×26.5 cm. (Evans 40143) (WU) **AIHP 03**

B4 The pharmacopoeia of the United States of America. By the authority of the Medical Societies and Colleges. Boston: Wells and Lilly, Printers, Dec. **1820**. 2 *l*, 5–272 p. 12×18 cm. (AIHP) **AIHP 58**

C16 PARIS, John Ayrton, 1785–1856

Pharmacologia; or the history of medicinal substances, with a view to establish the art of prescribing and of composing extemporaneous formulae upon fixed and scientific principles; illustrated by formulae, in which the intention of each element is designated by key letters. From the last London edition, with a general English index. New York: F. & R. Lockwood, **1822**. 1 *l*, iii–xii, 1 *l*, 15–428 p. 14×22 cm. (WU) **AIHP 48**

C29 THOMSON, Samuel, 1769–1843

New guide to health; or botanic family physician containing a complete system of practice, upon a plan entirely new; with a description of the vegetables made use of, and directions for preparing and administering them to cure disease. Boston: E. G. House, Printer, **1822**. 2 *l*, 184–300 p., 1 *l*; bound together with an Introduction written by a friend. 10×17.5 cm. (WU) **AIHP 73**

D4 The druggist's manual. Being a price current of drugs, medicines, paints, dye-stuffs, glass, patent medicines, etc., with Latin and English synonyms, a German, French, and Spanish catalogue of drugs, etc. Compiled by direction of the Philadelphia College of Pharmacy. Philadelphia: Solomon W. Conrad, Printer, **1826**. xvii, 119 p. 13.5×22 cm. (WU) **AIHP 12**

C17 RAFINESQUE, Constantine S[amuel], 1783–1840

Medical flora; or manual of the medical botany of the United States of North America. Two vols. in one. Philadelphia: Atkinson & Alexander, vol. 1 **1828**; vol. 2 **1830**. Vol. 1: 1 *l*, xii, 268 p. Vol. 2: 276 p. 10.5×18 cm. (DNLM) **AIHP 62**

A4 WOOD, George B., 1797–1879 and BACHE, Franklin, 1792–1864

The dispensatory of the United States of America. Philadelphia: Grigg & Elliot, **1833**. 1 *l*, v–x,1 *l*, 1073 p. 15×21 cm. (WU) **AIHP 82**

C18 DUNGLISON, Robley, 1798–1869

New remedies: the method of preparing and administering them; their effects on the healthy and diseased economy, &c. New York: Adam Waldie, **1839**. 3 *l*, i–viii, 429 p. 14×23 cm. (DNLM) **AIHP 13**

C30 PAINE, Martyn, 1794–1877

Essays on the philosophy of vitality . . . and on the modus operandi of remedial agents. New York: Hopkins & Jennings, Printer, **1842.** 2 *l*, v–viii, 2–70 p. 14.5×22.5 cm. (DNLM) **AIHP 46**

C19 PAINE, Martyn, 1794–1877

A therapeutical arrangement of the materia medica, or the materia medica arranged upon physiological principles, and in the order of the general practical value which remedial agents hold and their several denominations, and in conformity with the physiological doctrines set forth in the medical and physiological commentaries. New York: J. & H. G. Langley, **1842.** 2 *l*, vi–xii, 14–271 p. 11×18.5 cm. (WU) **AIHP 47**

C35 BECK, Lewis C[aleb], 1798–1853

Adulteration of various substances used in medicine and the arts with the means of detecting them. New York: Samuel S. and William Wood, **1846.** xi, 332 p. 12.5×20 cm. (DNLM) **AIHP 04**

C20 GRIFFITH, R. Eglesfeld, 1798–1850

Medical botany: or descriptions of the more important plants used in medicine, with their history, properties, and mode of administration. Philadelphia: Lea and Blanchard, **1847.** 2 *l*, vii–xv, [17]-704 p., 16 *l*. 15×23 cm. (WU) **AIHP 20**

C1   MOHR, Francis [Carl Friedrich], 1806–1879 and REDWOOD, Theophilus, 1806–1892

Practical pharmacy: The arrangements, apparatus, and manipulations, of the pharmaceutical shop and laboratory. Edited, with extensive additions, by William Procter, Jr., (1817–1874). Philadelphia: Lea and Blanchard, **1849.** xvi, 2, 18–576 p. 14×21 cm. (WU) **AIHP 38**

B5 GRIFFITH, R. Eglesfeld, 1798–1850

A universal formulary: containing the methods of preparing and administering officinal and other medicines. The whole adapted to physicians and pharmaceutists. Philadelphia: Lea and Blanchard, **1850.** 2 *l*, viii–ix, 9–567 p. 14.5×22.5 cm. (DNLM) **AIHP 21**

A5 KING, John, 1813–1893, and NEWTON, Robert S., 1818–1881

The eclectic dispensatory of the United States of America. Authorized by the Eclectic National Medical Convention. Cincinnati: H. W. Derby & Co., **1852.** 1 *l*, v–viii, 708 p. 14×21 cm. (WU) **AIHP 29**

C2 PARRISH, Edward, 1822–1872

An introduction to practical pharmacy. Designed as a text-book for the student and as a guide to the physician and pharmaceutist with many formulas and prescriptions. Philadelphia: Blanchard & Lea, **1856.** v–xxiv, 18–544 p. 14.5×22 cm. (WU) **AIHP 49**

D5 T. Morris Perot and Co.

Prices current for druggists only. Drugs, medicines, chemicals, etc. Philadelphia: no publ., [c. **1857** or c. **1858**] 52 p. 13×21 cm. (WU) **AIHP 51**

C46 Minutes of the convention of pharmaceutists and druggists held in the city of New York, October 15, 1851. Philadelphia: Merrihew & Son, Printers, **1865.** 1 *l*, 4–11 p. 14.5×21.5 cm. Bound together with "Proceedings of the National Pharmaceutical Convention held in Philadelphia, October 6th, 1852." Philadelphia: Merrihew & Son, Printers, (second unaltered edition) 1865. 2 *l*, 6–32 p.; "Proceedings of the American Pharmaceutical Association at the annual meeting, held in Boston, August 24th, 25th and 26th, 1853." Philadelphia: Merrihew & Thompson, Printers, 1853. 1 *l*, 4–48 p.; "Proceedings of the American Pharmaceutical Association at the third annual meeting, held in Cincinnati July 25th and 26th, 1854." Philadelphia, Merrihew & Thompson Printers, 1854. 1 *l*, 4–40 p.; "Proceedings of the American Pharmaceutical Association at the fourth annual meeting, held in New York, September 11th, 12th and 13th, 1855." Philadelphia: Merrihew & Son, Printers (second unaltered edition), 1865. 1 *l*, 4–40 p. (WU) **AIHP 36**

C40 MAISCH, John M[ichael], 1831–1893

Report on legislation regulating the practice of pharmacy in the United States. Philadelphia: Merrihew and Son, Printers, **1868**. 48 p. 14×22.5 cm. (WU) **AIHP 32**

C36 ATTFIELD, John, 1835–1911

Chemistry: general, medical and pharmaceutical. Philadelphia: Henry C. Lea, **1871**. iii–xi, 14–552 p. 11.5×18.5 cm. (WU) **AIHP 01**

D6 McKesson & Robbins (firm)

Prices current of drugs and druggists' articles, chemical and pharmaceutical preparations, proprietary medicines and perfumery, sponges, corks, dyes, paints, etc. New York: Thitchener and Glastaeter, Printers, **1872**. 3 *l*, 8–128 p. 14.5×21 cm. (WU) **AIHP 34**

C37 HOFFMANN, Frederick, 1832–1904

Manual of chemical analysis as applied to the examination of medicinal chemicals. A guide for the determination of their identity and quality, and for the detection of impurities and adulterations. For the use of pharmaceutists, physicians, druggists, and manufacturing chemists and of pharmaceutical and medical students. New York: D. Appleton & Co., **1873**. 1 *l*, iii, 8–393 p. 14.5×22.5 cm. (ICRL) **AIHP 25**

C3 SWERINGEN, H[iram] V., 1844–1912

Pharmaceutical lexicon: A dictionary of pharmaceutical science. Containing a concise explanation of the various subjects and terms of pharmacy ... designed as a guide for the pharmaceutist, druggist, physician, etc. Philadelphia: Lindsay & Blakiston, **1873**. vi, 576 p. 14×21 cm. (WU) **AIHP 71**

C31 HERING, C[onstantin], 1800–1880

Condensed materia medica, compiled with the assistance of Drs. A. Korndoerfer and E. A. Farrington. New York and Philadelphia: Boericke and Tafel, **1877.** 1 *l*, vii–xvi, 870 p., 1 *l.* 16×22 cm. (WU) **AIHP 23**

C21 RUDOLPHY, John

Chemical and pharmaceutical directory of all the chemicals and preparations (compound drugs) . . . in general use in the drug trade. Their names and synonyms alphabetically arranged. In three parts: I English, Latin and German names; II Latin, German and English names; III German, Latin and English names. Chicago: John Rudolphy, **1877.** 3 *l*, 8–407 p. 16×25 cm. (WU) **AIHP 67**

C22 RUDOLPHY, John

Pharmaceutical directory of all the crude drugs now in general use; their etymology and names in alphabetical order. In four parts: I English, botanical, pharmaceutical and German names; II Botanical, English, pharmaceutical and German names; III Pharmaceutical, botanical, English and German names; IV German, pharmaceutical, botanical and English names. Third edition. New York: William Radde, **1877.** 8, 2 *l*, 5–119 p. 17×26 cm. (WU) **AIHP 68**

C4 BOERICKE, F. E., b. 1829

Three lectures on homoeopathic pharmaceutics. New York and Philadelphia: Boericke and Tafel, [c. **1878**]. 1 *l*, 3–49 p. 13×21.5 cm. (WU) **AIHP 05**

B6 KILNER, Walter B., b. 1847

A compendium of modern pharmacy and druggists' formulary. Containing the recent methods of manufacturing and preparing elixirs, tinctures, fluid extracts, flavoring extracts, emulsions, perfumery and toilet articles, wines and liquors; also physician's prescriptions, liniments, pills, powders, ointments, syrups, antidotes to poisons, weights and measures, and miscellaneous information indispensible to the pharmacist. Springfield, IL: H. W. Rokker, Printer, **1880.** 1 *l*, 3–478 p. 13.5×18.5 cm. (DNLM) **AIHP 28**

D7 Whitall, Tatum and Co.

Glass manufacture. Druggists' sundries. Philadelphia and New York: no publ., **1880**. 72 p. 15.5×23 cm. (WU) **AIHP 78**

C24 MAISCH, John M[ichael], 1831–1893

A manual of organic materia medica. Being a guide to materia medica of the vegetable and animal kingdoms, for the use of students, druggists, pharmacists, and physicians. Philadelphia: Henry C. Lea's Son & Co., **1882**. 1 *l*, iv–xv, 26–459 p. 13×19.5 cm. (ICRL) **AIHP 33**

B7 The pharmacopoeia of the United States of America. Sixth decennial revision. By authority of the National Convention for Revising the Pharmacopoeia held at Washington, A.D. 1880. New York: William Wood & Co., **1882**. xli, 487 p. 14×22 cm. (WU) **AIHP 59**

C38 LYONS, A[lbert] B[rown], 1841–1926

Manual of practical pharmaceutical assaying, including details of the simplest and best methods of determining the strength of crude drugs and of galenical preparations. Designed especially for the use of the student and of the practical pharmacist. Detroit: D. O. Haynes & Co., **1886**. iii–vi, 7–154 p. 12.5×17 cm. (WU) **AIHP 31**

C5 REMINGTON, Joseph P[rice], 1847–1918

The practice of pharmacy: A treatise on the modes of making and dispensing officinal, unofficinal, and extemporaneous preparations, with descriptions of their properties, uses, and doses. Intended as a hand-book for pharmacists and physicians and a text-book for students. Philadelphia and London: J. B. Lippincott Co., **1886**. 1 *l*, 3–1080 p. 14×20.5 cm. (WU) **AIHP 63**

C25 FLÜCKIGER, Friedrich A., 1828–1894 and TSCHIRCH, Alexander, 1856–1939

The principles of pharmacognosy. An introduction to the study of the crude substances of the vegetable kingdom.

Translated from the second . . . revised German edition by Frederick B. Power. New York: William Wood & Co., **1887.** 1 *l*, iv–xvi, 294 p. 14.5×21.5 cm. (WU) **AIHP 18**

B8 The national formulary of unofficinal preparations. By authority of the American Pharmaceutical Association. n.p.: American Pharmaceutical Association, **1888.** ix, 176 p. 15×21 cm. (WU) **AIHP 41**

D8 James W. Tufts (firm)

Arctic soda water apparatus. Boston, [c. **1888**]. 2 *l*, 5–220 p. 18.5×24 cm. (WU) **AIHP 74**

B9 OLESON, Charles W[ilmot], d. 1906

Secret nostrums and systems of medicine. A book of formulas. Chicago: Oleson & Co., **1890.** 1 *l*, 3–206 p. 12×17.5 cm. (DNLM) **AIHP 45**

D9 Henry Heil Chemical Company

Illustrated catalogue and price-list of chemical and physical apparatus and instruments for laboratories, chemists, iron and steel works, smelters, . . . schools, colleges, universities, etc. St. Louis: no publ., [c. **1891**]. 2 *l*, 10–447 p. 16×24.5 cm. (WU) **AIHP 22**

C47 OLDBERG, Oscar, 1846–1913

A course of home study for pharmacists. First lessons in the study of pharmacy. Chicago: The Apothecaries' Company, [c. **1891**]. 3 *l*, v–xiv, 1 *l*, 523 p. 15×22 cm. (WU) **AIHP 44**

C41 WEDDERBURN, Alex J.

A compilation of the pharmacy and drug laws of the several states and territories. U.S. Department of Agriculture, Division of Chemistry, Bulletin No. 42. Washington, D.C.: Government Printing Office, **1894.** 1 *l*, 3–152 p. 14.5×22.5 cm. (WU) **AIHP 77**

C6 SCOVILLE, Wilbur L[incoln], 1865–1942

The art of compounding. A textbook for students and a reference book for pharmacists and the prescription counter. Philadelphia: P. Blakiston Son & Co., **1895**. 1 *l*, 5×264 p. 15×22.5 cm. (ICRL) **AIHP 69**

B10 EBERT, Albert E., 1840–1906 and HISS, A. Emil, b. 1866

The standard formulary. A collection of over four thousand formulas for pharmaceutical preparations, family remedies, toilet articles, and miscellaneous preparations especially adapted to the requirements of retail druggists. Chicago: G. P. Engelhard & Co., **1896**. 4 *l*, [11], 500 p. 15×22.5 cm. (WU) **AIHP 15**

B11 Pharmacopoeia of the American Institute of Homoeopathy. Published for the Committee on Pharmacopoeia of the American Institute of Homoeopathy. Boston: Otis Clapp and Son, Agents, **1897**. 2 *l*, 7–674 p. 15.5×22.5 cm. (WU) **AIHP 54**

C7 WALL, Otto A., 1846–1922

The prescription, therapeutically, pharmaceutically, grammatically and historically considered. Third edition. St. Louis: Aug. Gast Bank Note and Litho. Co., **1898**. 2 *l*, 211 p. 13.5×19 cm. (WU) **AIHP 76**

C32 CUSHNY, Arthur Robertson, 1866–1926

A textbook of pharmacology and therapeutics or the action of drugs in health and disease. Philadelphia and New York: Lea Brothers & Co., **1899**. 2 *l*, 6–730 p. 14.5×23 cm. (ICRL) **AIHP 10**

B12 HISS, A. Emil, b. 1866

Thesaurus of proprietary preparations and pharmaceutical specialties. Including "patent" medicines, proprietary pharmaceuticals, open-formula specialties, synthetic remedies, etc. Chicago: G. P. Englehard & Co., **1899**. 1 *l*, 4–279 p. 15×22.5 cm. (AIHP) **AIHP 24**

D10 Peter Van Schaack and Sons

Annual price current. Drugs, chemicals, medicines. Chicago: J. M. W. Jones Stationery and Printing Co., Printers, **1899.** 5 *l*, 7–1116 p. 11.5×18 cm. (WU) **AIHP 75**

C8 RUDDIMAN, Edsel A., 1864–1954

Incompatibilities in prescriptions for students in pharmacy and medicine and practicing pharmacists and physicians. New York: John Wiley & Sons; London: Chapman & Hall, **1899.** 1 *l*, 1 p., iii, 264 p. 13.5×20.5 cm. (WU) **AIHP 66**

B13 The pharmacopoeia of the German Hospital of the city of Philadelphia. Including formulas for all stock preparations and the average doses of all drugs, chemicals, and preparations usually dispensed at the German Hospital pharmacy. Philadelphia: Board of Trustees, **1902.** 1 *l*, 3–144 p. 8.5×16.5 cm. (WU) **AIHP 55**

C42 WILEY, Harley R., d. 1924

A treatise on pharmacal jurisprudence with a thesis on the law in general. San Francisco: The Hicks-Judd Co., **1904.** 3 *l*, 4–262 p. 12.5×19.5 cm. (WU) **AIHP 80**

B14 The pharmacopoeia of the United States of America. Eighth decennial revision. By authority of the United States Pharmacopoeial Convention held at Washington, A.D. 1900. Official from September 1st **1905.** Philadelphia: P. Blakiston's Son & Co. *l*, xxv, 692 p. 14×21 cm. (WU) **AIHP 60**

C23 The modern materia medica. The source, chemical and physical properties, therapeutic action, dosage, antidotes and incompatibles of all additions to the newer materia medica that are likely to be called for on prescriptions. New York: The Druggists Circular, **1906.** 2 *l*, 6–306 p. 12.5×18.5 cm. (WU) **AIHP 37**

C33 New and non-official remedies. A reprint from the *Journal of the American Medical Association* of the articles tentatively approved by the Council on Pharmacy and Chemistry of the American Medical Association. Chicago: Press of the American Medical Association, **1907**. 1 *l*, 4–160 p. 13×21 cm. (WU) **AIHP 42**

C9 REMINGTON, Joseph P[rice], 1847–1918

The practice of pharmacy: A treatise on the modes of making and dispensing officinal, unofficinal, and extemporaneous preparations, with descriptions of medicinal substances, their properties, uses and doses. Intended as a hand-book for pharmacists and physicians and a textbook for students. Fifth edition. Philadelphia and London: J. B. Lippincott Co., **1907**. 2 *l*, iii–xxv, 1541 p. 15×24 cm. (WU) **AIHP 64**

C43 KEBLER, Lyman F., 1863–1955

Drug legislation in the United States revised to July 15, 1908. U.S. Department of Agriculture, Bureau of Chemistry Bulletin No. 98 (revised). Part I. Washington, D.C.: Government Printing Office, **1909**. 2–343 p. 14.5×23 cm. (WU) **AIHP 27**

C48 The pharmaceutical syllabus. First edition recommended by the National Committee representing the boards and schools of pharmacy of the United States for the first syllabus period of August 1, 1910 to July 31, 1915. n.p.: J. B. Lyon Co., Printers, **1910**. 1 *l*, 4–146 p. 14.5×21.5 cm. (WU) **AIHP 53**

D11 M. Winter Lumber Company

Winter's Catalogue - No. 87. Commercial furniture; drug, jewelry and cigar store fixtures. Sheboygan, WI: no publ., **1910**. 1 *l*, B–Q, x, xx, 2 *l*, 320–629 p. 22.5×30 cm. (WU) **AIHP 81**

C44 WILBERT, Martin I., 1865–1916 and MOTTER, Murray Galt, 1866–1926

Digest of laws and regulations in force in the United States relating to the possession, use, sale, and manufacture of poisons and habit-forming drugs. United States Public Health Service, Public Health Bulletin No. 56. Washington, D.C.: Government Printing Office, **1912**. 1 *l*, 3–278 p. 15×23 cm. (WU) **AIHP 79**

C10 FANTUS, Bernard, 1874–1940

A text book on prescription-writing and pharmacy with practice in prescription-writing, laboratory exercises in pharmacy and a reference list of the official drugs especially designed for medical students. Second edition. Chicago: Chicago Medical Book Co., **1913**. iii–xii, 404 p. 14.5×22.5 cm. (WU) **AIHP 17**

C39 PITTENGER, Paul S., b. 1889

Biochemic drug assay methods with special reference to the pharmacodynamic standardization of drugs. Philadelphia: P. Blakiston's Son & Co., [c. **1914**]. 1 *l*, v–xv, 158 p. 13.5×17.5 cm. (WU) **AIHP 61**

C49 Year book of the American Pharmaceutical Association 1912. Scio, OH: The American Pharmaceutical Association, **1914**. 1 *l*, v–xl, 621 p. 14.5×22 cm. (WU) **AIHP 83**

B15 The druggists circular formula book. In which may be found recipes for hundreds of unofficial preparations in daily demand in the drugstore, the laboratory, the boudoir, the household . . .; together with a compilation of process outlines, notes, hints and other valuable information and suggestions for retail druggists and dispensing pharmacists culled from the pages of that publication. New York: The Druggists Circular, **1915**. 2 *l*, 5–242 p. 15×21 cm. (WU) **AIHP 11**

C26 KRAEMER, Henry, 1868-1924

Scientific and applied pharmacognosy. Intended for the use of students in pharmacy, as a handbook for pharmacists, and as a reference book for food and drug analysts and pharmacologists. Philadelphia: Published by the author, [c. **1915**]. v–viii, 857 p. 15×22 cm. (WU) **AIHP 30**

C34 SOLLMAN, Torald, 1874–1965

A manual of pharmacology and its applications to therapeutics and toxicology. Philadelphia and London: W. B. Saunders Company, **1917.** 1 *l*, 9–901 p. 16×23.5 cm. (WU)

D12 Wm. S. Merrell Company

Complete descriptive catalog of pharmaceutical preparations and ethical specialties. Cincinnati, [c. **1918**]. 1 *l*, 5–200 p. 12×19.5 cm. (WU) **AIHP 35**

C27 YOUNGKEN, Heber W[ilkinson], 1885–1963

A text book of pharmacognosy. Philadelphia: P. Blakiston's Son & Co., [c. **1921**]. 1 *l*, v–x, 1 *l*, 3–538 p. 15×23 cm. (DNLM) **AIHP 85**

A6 WOOD, Horatio C., Jr., 1874–1958 and LAWALL, Charles H., 1871–1937

The dispensatory of the United States of America. Twenty-first edition. Philadelphia and London: J. B. Lippincott Co., [c. **1926**]. 3 *l*, iii–xxx, 1792 p. 17.5×25.5 cm. (WU)

C50 CHARTERS, W[erret] W[allace] et al., 1875–1952

Basic material for a pharmaceutical curriculum. New York and London: McGraw-Hill Book Co., Inc., **1927.** xiii, 366 p. 14×22 cm. (WU) **AIHP 07**

C51 National Conference on Pharmaceutical Research, **1928/ 29–1932/33.** No place or date of publication. 372 p. Each year numbered separately. 13.5×20.5 cm. (WU) **AIHP 40**

B16 The pharmaceutical recipe book. By authority of the American Pharmaceutical Association. n.p.: The American Pharmaceutical Association, **1929.** iii–vii, 454 p. 15×22.5 cm. (WU) **AIHP 52**

C52 ROREM, C[larence] Rufus, b. 1894 and FISCHELIS, Robert P., 1891–1981

The costs of medicines. The manufacture and distribution of drugs and medicines in the United States and the services of pharmacy in medical care. Publication No. 14 of the Committee on the Costs of Medical Care. Chicago: University of Chicago Press, [c. **1932**]. xi, 250 p., 3 *l.* 15×21 cm. (WU) **AIHP 65**

C53 GATHERCOAL, E[dmund] N[orris], 1874–1954

The prescription ingredient survey. Consisting of: The Ebert survey 1885; Hallberg survey 1895; Hallberg-Snow survey 1907; Charters survey 1926; Cook survey 1930; Gathercoal survey 1930; U.S.P.-N.F. survey 1931–32. n.p.: The American Pharmaceutical Association, **1933**. 172 p. 17×25 cm. (WU) **AIHP 19**

C11 HUSA, William J., 1896–1985

Pharmaceutical dispensing. A textbook for students of pharmaceutical compounding and dispensing. Easton, PA: Mack Printing Co., Printers, **1935**. 1 *l*, v–vii, 1 *l*, 428 p. 15×21 cm. (WU) **AIHP 26**

C54 Year book of the American Pharmaceutical Association 1934. Washington, D.C.: American Pharmaceutical Association, **1936**. 1 *l*, xxxix, 1 *l*, 3–468 p. 14.5×22 cm. (WU) **AIHP 84**

C45 O'CONNELL, C. Leonard, 1890–1958 and PETTIT, William, 1907–1982

A manual on pharmaceutical law. Together with appendices containing important laws of Congress, the uniform narcotic drug law, and other laws relating to pharmacy. Philadelphia: Lea Febiger, **1938**. 2 *l*, 6–196 p. 13.5×20 cm. (WU) **AIHP 43**

D13 S. B. Penick & Company

Price list and manual of botanical crude drugs from the four corners of the earth. New York and Chicago, August 1, **1938**. 48 p. 11×19.5 cm. (WU) **AIHP 50**

PART THREE: ALPHABETICAL LIST OF SOURCES BY AUTHORS

C36 ATTFIELD, John, 1835–1911

Chemistry: general, medical and pharmaceutical. Philadelphia: Henry C. Lea, 1871. iii–xi, 14–552 p. 11.5×18.5 cm. (WU) **AIHP 01**

C14 BARTON, Benjamin Smith, 1766–1815

Collections for an essay towards a materia medica of the United States. Third edition. Philadelphia: Edward Earle and Co., 1810. Part first: 2 *l*, v–xvi, 3–67 p. Part second: 1 *l*, iii–xv, 53 p. 12.5×21 cm. (Evans 19478) (WU) **AIHP 02**

C15 BARTON, William P[aul] C[rillon], 1786–1856

Vegetable materia medica of the United States, or medical botany: containing a botanical, general, and medical history of medicinal plants indigenous to the United States. Illustrated by coloured engravings made after original drawings from nature, done by the author. Two vols. Philadelphia: M. Carey & Son, vol. 1 1817; vol. 2 1818. Vol. 1: 3 *l*, vi–xv, 17–273 p. 21×26.5 cm. Vol 2: 3 *l*, viii–xvi, 9–243 p. 21×26.5 cm. (Evans 40143) (WU) **AIHP 03**

C35 BECK, Lewis C[aleb], 1798–1853

Adulteration of various substances used in medicine and the arts with the means of detecting them. New York: Samuel S. and William Wood, 1846. xi, 332 p. 12.5×20 cm. (DNLM) **AIHP 04**

C4 BOERICKE, F. E., b. 1829

Three lectures on homoeopathic pharmaceutics. New York and Philadelphia: Boericke and Tafel, [c. 1878]. 1 *l*, 3–49 p. 13×21.5 cm. (WU) **AIHP 05**

107

B1 [BROWN, William], 1748-1792

Pharmacopoeia simpliciorum et efficaciorum in usum nosocomii militaris. Philadelphia: Styner & Cist., 1778. 4–32 p. 9.5×16 cm. (Evans 15750) (DNLM) **AIHP 06**

C50 CHARTERS, W[erret] W[allace] et al., 1875-1952

Basic material for a pharmaceutical curriculum. New York and London: McGraw-Hill Book Co., Inc., 1927. xiii, 366 p. 14×22 cm. (WU) **AIHP 07**

C12 CULLEN, William, 1710-1790

Lectures on the materia medica as delivered by William Cullen, M.D., professor of medicine in the University of Edinburgh. Now published by permission of the author, and with many corrections from the collation of different manuscripts by the editors. Philadelphia: Robert Bell, Printer, 1775. viii, 512 p. 19×24 cm. (Evans 14000) (WU) **AIHP 08**

A1 CULPEPER, Nicholas, 1616-1654

Pharmacopoeia Londinensis; or, the London dispensatory further adorned by the studies and collections of the fellows now living of the said college. Boston: John Allen, Printer, 1720. [24], 305 p., [35]. 11.5×18.5 cm. (Evans 2114) (DNLM) **AIHP 09**

C32 CUSHNY, Arthur Robertson, 1866-1926

A textbook of pharmacology and therapeutics or the action of drugs in health and disease. Philadelphia and New York: Lea Brothers & Co., 1899. 2 *l*, 6-730 p. 14.5×23 cm. (ICRL) **AIHP 10**

D1 John Day and Co.

Catalogue of drugs, chymical and galenical preparations, shop furniture, patent medicines, and surgeon instruments ... Philadelphia: John Dunlap, Printer, 1771. 29 p. (Evans 12024) (PPAmP)

B15 The druggists circular formula book. In which may be found recipes for hundreds of unofficial preparations in daily demand in the drugstore, the laboratory, the boudoir, the household . . .; together with a compilation of process outlines, notes, hints and other valuable information and suggestions for retail druggists and dispensing pharmacists culled from the pages of that publication. New York: The Druggists Circular, 1915. 2 *l*, 5–242 p. 15×21 cm. (WU) **AIHP 11**

D4 The druggist's manual. Being a price current of drugs, medicines, paints, dye-stuffs, glass, patent medicines, etc., with Latin and English synonyms, a German, French, and Spanish catalogue of drugs, etc. Compiled by direction of the Philadelphia College of Pharmacy. Philadelphia: Solomon W. Conrad, Printer, 1826. xvii, 119 p. 13.5×22 cm. (WU) **AIHP 12**

C18 DUNGLISON, Robley, 1798–1869

New remedies: the method of preparing and administering them; their effects on the healthy and diseased economy, &c. New York: Adam Waldie, 1839. 3 *l*, i–viii, 429 p. 14×23 cm. (DNLM) **AIHP 13**

D3 T[homas] W. Dyott (firm)

Approved patent and family medicines, which are celebrated for the cure of most diseases to which the human body is liable . . . for sale in Philadelphia only at the proprietors wholesale and retail drug and family medicine warehouse . . . Philadelphia, 1814. 28 p. 13.5×21.5 cm. (Evans 31384) (WU) **AIHP 14**

B10 EBERT, Albert E., 1840–1906 and HISS, A. Emil, b. 1866

The standard formulary. A collection of over four thousand formulas for pharmaceutical preparations, family remedies, toilet articles, and miscellaneous preparations especially adapted to the requirements of retail druggists. Chicago: G. P. Engelhard & Co., 1896. 4 *l*, [11], 500 p. 15×22.5 cm. (WU) **AIHP 15**

A2 The Edinburgh new dispensatory. Containing I The Elements of pharmaceutical chemistry. II The Materia medica. III The Pharmaceutical and medicinal compositions of the new editions of the London (1788) and Edinburgh (1783) pharmacopoeias. Philadelphia: T. Dobson, Printer, 1791. 3 *l*, vii–xxii, 33–656 p. 12.5×20 cm. (Evans 23503) (WU) **AIHP 16**

C10 FANTUS, Bernard, 1874–1940

A text book on prescription-writing and pharmacy with practice in prescription-writing, laboratory exercises in pharmacy and a reference list of the official drugs especially designed for medical students. Second edition. Chicago: Chicago Medical Book Co., 1913. iii–xii, 404 p. 14.5×22.5 cm. (WU) **AIHP 17**

C25 FLÜCKIGER, Friedrich A., 1828–1894 and TSCHIRCH, Alexander, 1856–1939

The principles of pharmacognosy. An introduction to the study of the crude substances of the vegetable kingdom. Translated from the second . . . revised German edition by Frederick B. Power. New York: William Wood & Co., 1887. 1 *l*, iv–xvi, 294 p. 14.5×21.5 cm. (WU) **AIHP 18**

C53 GATHERCOAL, E[dmund] N[orris], 1874–1954

The prescription ingredient survey. Consisting of: The Ebert survey 1885; Hallberg survey 1895; Hallberg-Snow survey 1907; Charters survey 1926; Cook survey 1930; Gathercoal survey 1930; U.S.P.-N.F. survey 1931–32. n.p.: The American Pharmaceutical Association, 1933. 172 p. 17×25 cm. (WU) **AIHP 19**

C20 GRIFFITH, R. Eglesfeld, 1798–1850

Medical botany: or descriptions of the more important plants used in medicine, with their history, properties, and mode of administration. Philadelphia: Lea and Blanchard, 1847. 2 *l*, vii–xv, [17]–704 p., 16 *l*. 15×23 cm. (WU) **AIHP 20**

B5 GRIFFITH, R. Eglesfeld, 1798–1850

A universal formulary: containing the methods of preparing and administering officinal and other medicines. The whole adapted to physicians and pharmaceutists. Philadelphia: Lea and Blanchard, 1850. 2 *l*, viii–ix, 9–567 p. 14.5×22.5 cm. (DNLM) **AIHP 21**

D9 Henry Heil Chemical Company

Illustrated catalogue and price-list of chemical and physical apparatus and instruments for laboratories, chemists, iron and steel works, smelters, . . . schools, colleges, universities, etc. St. Louis: no publ., [c. 1891]. 2 *l*, 10–447 p. 16×24.5 cm. (WU) **AIHP 22**

C31 HERING, C[onstantin], 1800–1880

Condensed materia medica, compiled with the assistance of Drs. A. Korndoerfer and E. A. Farrington. New York and Philadelphia: Boericke and Tafel, 1877. 1 *l*, vii–xvi, 870 p., 1 *l*. 16×22 cm. (WU) **AIHP 23**

B12 HISS, A. Emil, b. 1866

Thesaurus of proprietary preparations and pharmaceutical specialties. Including "patent" medicines, proprietary pharmaceuticals, open-formula specialties, synthetic remedies, etc. Chicago: G. P. Englehard & Co., 1899. 1 *l*, 4–279 p. 15×22.5 cm. (AIHP) **AIHP 24**

C37 HOFFMANN, Frederick, 1832–1904

Manual of chemical analysis as applied to the examination of medicinal chemicals. A guide for the determination of their identity and quality, and for the detection of impurities and adulterations. For the use of pharmaceutists, physicians, druggists, and manufacturing chemists and of pharmaceutical and medical students. New York: D. Appleton & Co., 1873. 1 *l*, iii, 8–393 p. 14.5×22.5 cm. (ICRL) **AIHP 25**

C11 HUSA, William J., 1896–1985

Pharmaceutical dispensing. A textbook for students of pharmaceutical compounding and dispensing. Easton, PA: Mack Printing Co., Printers, 1935. 1 *l*, v–vii, 1 *l*, 428 p. 15×21 cm. (WU) **AIHP 26**

C43 KEBLER, Lyman F., 1863–1955

Drug legislation in the United States revised to July 15, 1908. U.S. Department of Agriculture, Bureau of Chemistry Bulletin No. 98 (revised). Part I. Washington, D.C.: Government Printing Office, 1909. 2–343 p. 14.5×23 cm. (WU) **AIHP 27**

B6 KILNER, Walter B., b. 1847

A compendium of modern pharmacy and druggists' formulary. Containing the recent methods of manufacturing and preparing elixirs, tinctures, fluid extracts, flavoring extracts, emulsions, perfumery and toilet articles, wines and liquors; also physician's prescriptions, liniments, pills, powders, ointments, syrups, antidotes to poisons, weights and measures, and miscellaneous information indispensible to the pharmacist. Springfield, IL: H. W. Rokker, Printer, 1880. 1 *l*, 3–478 p. 13.5×18.5 cm. (DNLM) **AIHP 28**

A5 KING, John, 1813–1893, and NEWTON, Robert S., 1818–1881

The eclectic dispensatory of the United States of America. Authorized by the Eclectic National Medical Convention. Cincinnati: H. W. Derby & Co., 1852. 1 *l*, v–viii, 708 p. 14×21 cm. (WU) **AIHP 29**

C26 KRAEMER, Henry, 1868–1924

Scientific and applied pharmacognosy. Intended for the use of students in pharmacy, as a handbook for pharmacists, and as a reference book for food and drug analysts and pharmacologists. Philadelphia: Published by the author, [c. 1915]. v–viii, 857 p. 15×22 cm. (WU) **AIHP 30**

C38 LYONS, A[lbert] B[rown], 1841–1926

Manual of practical pharmaceutical assaying, including details of the simplest and best methods of determining the strength of crude drugs and of galenical preparations. Designed especially for the use of the student and of the practical pharmacist. Detroit: D. O. Haynes & Co., 1886. iii–vi, 7–154 p. 12.5×17 cm. (WU) **AIHP 31**

C40 MAISCH, John M[ichael], 1831–1893

Report on legislation regulating the practice of pharmacy in the United States. Philadelphia: Merrihew and Son, Printers, 1868. 48 p. 14×22.5 cm. (WU) **AIHP 32**

C24 MAISCH, John M[ichael], 1831–1893

A manual of organic materia medica. Being a guide to materia medica of the vegetable and animal kingdoms, for the use of students, druggists, pharmacists, and physicians. Philadelphia: Henry C. Lea's Son & Co., 1882. 1 *l*, iv–xv, 26–459 p. 13×19.5 cm. (ICRL) **AIHP 33**

D6 McKesson & Robbins (firm)

Prices current of drugs and druggists' articles, chemical and pharmaceutical preparations, proprietary medicines and perfumery, sponges, corks, dyes, paints, etc. New York: Thitchener and Glastaeter, Printers, 1872. 3 *l*, 8–128 p. 14.5×21 cm. (WU) **AIHP 34**

D12 Wm. S. Merrell Company

Complete descriptive catalog of pharmaceutical preparations and ethical specialties. Cincinnati, [c. 1918]. 1 *l*, 5–200 p. 12×19.5 cm. (WU) **AIHP 35**

C46 Minutes of the convention of pharmaceutists and druggists held in the city of New York, October 15, 1851. Philadelphia: Merrihew & Son, Printers, 1865. 1 *l*, 4–11 p. 14.5×21.5 cm. Bound together with "Proceedings of the National Pharmaceutical Convention held in Philadelphia, October 6th, 1852." Philadelphia: Merrihew & Son, Printers, (second unaltered edition) 1865. 2 *l*, 6–32 p.; "Proceedings of the American Pharmaceutical Association at the annual meeting, held in Boston, August 24th, 25th and 26th, 1853." Philadelphia: Merrihew & Thompson, Printers, 1853. 1 *l*, 4–48 p.; "Proceedings of the American Pharmaceutical Association at the third annual meeting, held in Cincinnati July 25th and 26th, 1854." Philadelphia, Merrihew & Thompson Printers, 1854. 1 *l*, 4–40 p.; "Proceedings of the American Pharmaceutical Association at the fourth annual meeting, held in New York, September 11th, 12th and 13th, 1855." Philadelphia: Merrihew & Son, Printers (second unaltered edition), 1865. 1 *l*, 4–40 p. (WU) **AIHP 36**

C23 The modern materia medica. The source, chemical and physical properties, therapeutic action, dosage, antidotes and incompatibles of all additions to the newer materia medica that are likely to be called for on prescriptions. New York: The Druggists Circular, 1906. 2 *l*, 6–306 p. 12.5×18.5 cm. (WU) **AIHP 37**

C1 MOHR, Francis [Carl Friedrich], 1806–1879 and REDWOOD, Theophilus, 1806–1892

Practical pharmacy: The arrangements, apparatus, and manipulations, of the pharmaceutical shop and laboratory. Edited, with extensive additions, by William Procter, Jr., (1817–1874). Philadelphia: Lea and Blanchard, 1849. xvi, 2, 18–576 p. 14×21 cm. (WU) **AIHP 38**

C13 MURRAY, J[ohn], 1778–1820

Elements of materia medica and pharmacy. Two vols. in one. Philadelphia: B. and T. Kite, 1808. vi–xii, 13–447 p. 12.5×20 cm. (Evans 15670) (WU) **AIHP 39**

C51 National Conference on Pharmaceutical Research, 1928/29–1932/33. No place or date of publication. 372 p. Each year numbered separately. 13.5×20.5 cm. (WU) **AIHP 40**

B8 The national formulary of unofficinal preparations. By authority of the American Pharmaceutical Association. n.p.: American Pharmaceutical Association, 1888. ix, 176 p. 15×21 cm. (WU) **AIHP 41**

C33 New and non-official remedies. A reprint from the *Journal of the American Medical Association* of the articles tentatively approved by the Council on Pharmacy and Chemistry of the American Medical Association. Chicago: Press of the American Medical Association, 1907. 1 *l*, 4160 p. 13×21 cm. (WU) **AIHP 42**

C45 O'CONNELL, C. Leonard, 1890–1958 and PETTIT, William, 1907–1982

A manual on pharmaceutical law. Together with appendices containing important laws of Congress, the uniform narcotic drug law, and other laws relating to pharmacy. Philadelphia: Lea Febiger, 1938. 2 *l*, 6–196 p. 13.5×20 cm. (WU) **AIHP 43**

C47 OLDBERG, Oscar, 1846–1913

A course of home study for pharmacists. First lessons in the study of pharmacy. Chicago: The Apothecaries' Company, [c. 1891]. 3 *l*, v–xiv, 1 *l*, 523 p. 15×22 cm. (WU) **AIHP 44**

B9 OLESON, Charles W[ilmot], d. 1906

Secret nostrums and systems of medicine. A book of formulas. Chicago: Oleson & Co., 1890. 1 *l*, 3–206 p. 12×17.5 cm. (DNLM) **AIHP 45**

C30 PAINE, Martyn, 1794–1877

Essays on the philosophy of vitality . . . and on the modus operandi of remedial agents. New York: Hopkins & Jennings, Printer, 1842. 2 *l*, v–viii, 2–70 p. 14.5×22.5 cm. (DNLM) **AIHP 46**

C19 PAINE, Martyn, 1794–1877

A therapeutical arrangement of the materia medica, or the materia medica arranged upon physiological principles, and in the order of the general practical value which remedial agents hold and their several denominations, and in conformity with the physiological doctrines set forth in the medical and physiological commentaries. New York: J. & H. G. Langley, 1842. 2 *l*, vi–xii, 14–271 p. 11×18.5 cm. (WU) **AIHP 47**

C16 PARIS, John Ayrton, 1785–1856

Pharmacologia; or the history of medicinal substances, with a view to establish the art of prescribing and of composing extemporaneous formulae upon fixed and scientific principles; illustrated by formulae, in which the intention of each element is designated by key letters. From the last London edition, with a general English index. New York: F. & R. Lockwood, 1822. 1 *l*, iii–xii, 1 *l*, 15–428 p. 14×22 cm. (WU) **AIHP 48**

C2 PARRISH, Edward, 1822–1872

An introduction to practical pharmacy. Designed as a text-book for the student and as a guide to the physician and pharmaceutist with many formulas and prescriptions. Philadelphia: Blanchard & Lea, 1856. v–xxiv, 18–544 p. 14.5×22 cm. (WU) **AIHP 49**

D13 S. B. Penick & Company

Price list and manual of botanical crude drugs from the four corners of the earth. New York and Chicago, August 1, 1938. 48 p. 11×19.5 cm. (WU) **AIHP 50**

D5 T. Morris Perot and Co.

Prices current for druggists only. Drugs, medicines, chemicals, etc. Philadelphia: no publ., [c. 1857 or c. 1858] 52 p. 13×21 cm. (WU) **AIHP 51**

B16 The pharmaceutical recipe book. By authority of the American Pharmaceutical Association. n.p.: The American Pharmaceutical Association, 1929. iii–vii, 454 p. 15×22.5 cm. (WU) **AIHP 52**

C48 The pharmaceutical syllabus. First edition recommended by the National Committee representing the boards and schools of pharmacy of the United States for the first syllabus period of August 1, 1910 to July 31, 1915. n.p.: J. B. Lyon Co., Printers, 1910. 1 *l*, 4–146 p. 14.5×21.5 cm. (WU) **AIHP 53**

B11 Pharmacopoeia of the American Institute of Homoeopathy. Published for the Committee on Pharmacopoeia of the American Institute of Homoeopathy. Boston: Otis Clapp and Son, Agents, 1897. 2 *l*, 7–674 p. 15.5×22.5 cm. (WU) **AIHP 54**

B13 The pharmacopoeia of the German Hospital of the city of Philadelphia. Including formulas for all stock preparations and the average doses of all drugs, chemicals, and preparations usually dispensed at the German Hospital pharmacy. Philadelphia: Board of Trustees, 1902. 1 *l*, 3–144 p. 8.5×16.5 cm. (WU) **AIHP 55**

B2 The pharmacopoeia of the Massachusetts Medical Society. Boston: E. & J. Larkin, 1808. 3 *l*, v–x, 2 *l*, 3–272 p. 10×18 cm. (Evans 15554) (WU) **AIHP 56**

B3 Pharmacopoeia nosocomii Neo-Eboracensis; or the pharmacopoeia of the New York Hospital . . . an appendix containing a general posological table and a comparative view of the former and present terms in materia medica and pharmacy. New York: Collins & Co., 1816. 2 *l*, vi–x, 1 *l*, 180, 1 p. 12×20 cm. (Evans 38453) (WU) **AIHP 57**

B4 The pharmacopoeia of the United States of America. By the authority of the Medical Societies and Colleges. Boston: Wells and Lilly, Printers, Dec. 1820. 2 *l*, 5–272 p. 12×18 cm. (AIHP) **AIHP 58**

B7   The pharmacopoeia of the United States of America. Sixth decennial revision. By authority of the National Convention for Revising the Pharmacopoeia held at Washington, A.D. 1880. New York: William Wood & Co., 1882. xli, 487 p. 14×22 cm. (WU) **AIHP 59**

B14 The pharmacopoeia of the United States of America. Eighth decennial revision. By authority of the United States Pharmacopoeial Convention held at Washington, A.D. 1900. Official from September 1st 1905. Philadelphia: P. Blakiston's Son & Co. *l*, xxv, 692 p. 14×21 cm. (WU) **AIHP 60**

C39 PITTENGER, Paul S., b. 1889

Biochemic drug assay methods with special reference to the pharmacodynamic standardization of drugs. Philadelphia: P. Blakiston's Son & Co., [c. 1914]. 1 *l*, v–xv, 158 p. 13.5×17.5 cm. (WU) **AIHP 61**

C17 RAFINESQUE, Constantine S[amuel], 1783–1840

Medical flora; or manual of the medical botany of the United States of North America. Two vols. in one. Philadelphia: Atkinson & Alexander, vol. 1 1828; vol. 2 1830. Vol. 1: 1 *l*, xii, 268 p. Vol. 2: 276 p. 10.5×18 cm. (DNLM) **AIHP 62**

C5   REMINGTON, Joseph P[rice], 1847–1918

The practice of pharmacy: A treatise on the modes of making and dispensing officinal, unofficinal, and extemporaneous preparations, with descriptions of their properties, uses, and doses. Intended as a hand-book for pharmacists and physicians and a text-book for students. Philadelphia and London: J. B. Lippincott Co., 1886. 1 *l*, 3–1080 p. 14×20.5 cm. (WU) **AIHP 63**

C9   REMINGTON, Joseph P[rice], 1847–1918

The practice of pharmacy: A treatise on the modes of making and dispensing officinal, unofficinal, and extemporaneous preparations, with descriptions of medicinal substances, their properties, uses and doses. Intended as a hand-book for pharmacists and physicians and a text-book for students. Fifth edition. Philadelphia and London: J. B. Lippincott Co., 1907. 2 *l*, iii–xxv, 1541 p. 15×24 cm. (WU) **AIHP 64**

C52 ROREM, C[larence] Rufus, b. 1894 and FISCHELIS, Robert P., 1891–1981

The costs of medicines. The manufacture and distribution of drugs and medicines in the United States and the services of pharmacy in medical care. Publication No. 14 of the Committee on the Costs of Medical Care. Chicago: University of Chicago Press, [c. 1932]. xi, 250 p., 3 *l*. 15×21 cm. (WU) **AIHP 65**

C8 RUDDIMAN, Edsel A., 1864–1954

Incompatibilities in prescriptions for students in pharmacy and medicine and practicing pharmacists and physicians. New York: John Wiley & Sons; London: Chapman & Hall, 1899. 1 *l*, 1 p. iii, 264 p. 13.5×20.5 cm. (WU) **AIHP 66**

C21 RUDOLPHY, John

Chemical and pharmaceutical directory of all the chemicals and preparations (compound drugs) . . . in general use in the drug trade. Their names and synonyms alphabetically arranged. In three parts: I English, Latin and German names; II Latin, German and English names; III German, Latin and English names. Chicago: John Rudolphy, 1877. 3 *l*, 8–407 p. 16×25 cm. (WU) **AIHP 67**

C22 RUDOLPHY, John

Pharmaceutical directory of all the crude drugs now in general use; their etymology and names in alphabetical order. In four parts: I English, botanical, pharmaceutical and German names; II Botanical, English, pharmaceutical and German names; III Pharmaceutical, botanical, English and German names; IV German, pharmaceutical, botanical and English names. Third edition. New York: William Radde, 1877. 8, 2 *l*, 5–119 p. 17×26 cm. (WU) **AIHP 68**

C6   SCOVILLE, Wilbur L[incoln], 1865–1942

The art of compounding. A textbook for students and a reference book for pharmacists and the prescription counter. Philadelphia: P. Blakiston Son & Co., 1895. 1 *l*, 5–264 p. 15×22.5 cm. (ICRL) **AIHP 69**

D2   Smith and Bartlett (firm)

Catalogue of drugs and medicines, instruments and utensils, dye-stuffs, groceries and painters' colours, imported, prepared, and sold by Smith & Bartlett at their druggists stores and apothecaries shop, Boston. Boston: Manning & Loring, Printers, 1795. 22 p. 11×17.5 cm. (Evans 29537) (MBCP) **AIHP 70**

C28   SMITH, Peter, 1753–1816

Indian doctor's dispensatory, being Father Smith's advice respecting diseases and their cure; consisting of prescriptions for many complaints; and a description of medicines, simple and compound, showing their virtues and how to apply them. Designed for the benefit of his children, his friends and the public, but more especially the citizens of the United States of America. Cincinnati: Browne and Looker, Printers, 1813. i-iv, 108 p. 17.1×10 cm. (OCLloyd)

C34   SOLLMAN, Torald, 1874–1965

A manual of pharmacology and its applications to therapeutics and toxicology. Philadelphia and London: W. B. Saunders Company, 1917. 1 *l*, 9–901 p. 16×23.5 cm. (WU)

C3   SWERINGEN, H[iram] V., 1844–1912

Pharmaceutical lexicon: A dictionary of pharmaceutical science. Containing a concise explanation of the various subjects and terms of pharmacy . . . designed as a guide for the pharmaceutist, druggist, physician, etc. Philadelphia: Lindsay & Blakiston, 1873. vi, 576 p. 14×21 cm. (WU) **AIHP 71**

A3 THACHER, James, 1754–1844

The American new dispensatory. Containing general principles of pharmaceutic chemistry. Pharmaceutic operations. Chemical analysis of the articles of materia medica. Materia medica including several new and valuable articles, the production of the United States. Preparations and compositions . . . . Boston: T. B. Wait & Co., 1810. 3 *l*, 7–529 p. 13×20 cm. (Evans 21476) (WU) **AIHP 72**

C29 THOMSON, Samuel, 1769–1843

New guide to health; or botanic family physician containing a complete system of practice, upon a plan entirely new; with a description of the vegetables made use of, and directions for preparing and administering them to cure disease. Boston: E. G. House, Printer, 1822. 2 *l*, 184–300 p., 1 *l*; bound together with an Introduction by a friend. 10×17.5 cm. (WU) **AIHP 73**

D8 James W. Tufts (firm)

Arctic soda water apparatus. Boston, [c. 1888]. 2 *l*, 5–220 p. 18.5×24 cm. (WU) **AIHP 74**

D10 Peter Van Schaack and Sons

Annual price current. Drugs, chemicals, medicines. Chicago: J. M. W. Jones Stationery and Printing Co., Printers, 1899. 5 *l*, 7–1116 p. 11.5×18 cm. (WU) **AIHP 75**

C7 WALL, Otto A., 1846–1922

The prescription, therapeutically, pharmaceutically, grammatically and historically considered. Third edition. St. Louis: Aug. Gast Bank Note and Litho. Co., 1898. 2 *l*, 211 p. 13.5×19 cm. (WU) **AIHP 76**

C41 WEDDERBURN, Alex J.

A compilation of the pharmacy and drug laws of the several states and territories. U.S. Department of Agriculture, Division of Chemistry, Bulletin No. 42. Washington, D.C.: Government Printing Office, 1894. 1 *l*, 3–152 p. 14.5×22.5 cm. (WU) **AIHP 77**

D7 Whitall, Tatum and Co.

Glass manufacture. Druggists' sundries. Philadelphia and New York: no publ., 1880. 72 p. 15.5×23 cm. (WU) **AIHP 78**

C44 WILBERT, Martin I., 1865–1916 and MOTTER, Murray Galt, 1866–1926

Digest of laws and regulations in force in the United States relating to the possession, use, sale, and manufacture of poisons and habit-forming drugs. United States Public Health Service, Public Health Bulletin No. 56. Washington, D.C.: Government Printing Office, 1912. 1 *l*, 3–278 p. 15×23 cm. (WU) **AIHP 79**

C42 WILEY, Harley R., d. 1924

A treatise on pharmacal jurisprudence with a thesis on the law in general. San Francisco: The Hicks-Judd Co., 1904. 3 *l*, 4–262 p. 12.5×19.5 cm. (WU) **AIHP 80**

D11 M. Winter Lumber Company

Winter's Catalogue - No. 87. Commercial furniture; drug, jewelry and cigar store fixtures. Sheboygan, WI: no publ., 1910. 1 *l*, B–Q, x, xx, 2 *l*, 320–629 p. 22.5×30 cm. (WU) **AIHP 81**

A4 WOOD, George B., 1797–1879 and BACHE, Franklin, 1792–1864

The dispensatory of the United States of America. Philadelphia: Grigg & Elliot, 1833. 1 *l*, v–x,1 *l*, 1073 p. 15×21 cm. (WU) **AIHP 82**

A6 WOOD, Horatio C., Jr., 1874–1958 and LAWALL, Charles H., 1871–1937

The dispensatory of the United States of America. Twenty-first edition. Philadelphia and London: J. B. Lippincott Co., [c. 1926]. 3 *l*, iii–xxx, 1792 p. 17.5×25.5 cm. (WU)

C49 Year book of the American Pharmaceutical Association 1912. Scio, OH: The American Pharmaceutical Association, 1914. 1 *l*, v–xl, 621 p. 14.5×22 cm. (WU) **AIHP 83**

C54 Year book of the American Pharmaceutical Association 1934. Washington, D.C.: American Pharmaceutical Association, 1936. 1 *l*, xxxix, 1 *l*, 3–468 p. 14.5×22 cm. (WU) **AIHP 84**

C27 YOUNGKEN, Heber W[ilkinson], 1885–1963

A text book of pharmacognosy. Philadelphia: P. Blakiston's Son & Co., [c. 1921]. 1 *l*, v–x, 1 *l*, 3–538 p. 15×23 cm. (DNLM) **AIHP 85**